SAFETY IN THE ARTROOM

SAFETY IN THE ARTROOM

CHARLES A. QUALLEY

Professor of Art, University of Colorado

Davis Publications, Inc., Worcester, Massachusetts

For my best friends, BJ, JL, and JS.

This book was written to provide the most current and accurate information available about health and safety hazards in art classrooms. However, the author and publisher can take no responsibility for any harm or damage that might be caused by the use or misuse of any information contained herein. It is not the purpose of this book to provide medical diagnosis or information, or to set health or safety standards for any art classroom. Readers should seek advice from physicians, safety professionals or environmental health specialists concerning specific problems and should in all cases carefully read and follow product information and instructions describing safe-use practices. Questions about specific products should be directed to the manufacturer.

Copyright 1986
Davis Publications, Inc.
Worcester, Massachusetts U.S.A.

PRINTED IN THE UNITED STATES OF AMERICA
Library of Congress Catalog Card Number: 85-073421
ISBN: 0-87192-174-X
10 9 8 7 6 5 4
DESIGNER and ILLUSTRATOR: George Lallas

ACKNOWLEDGMENTS

Ray Hall and David Baker are nearly as responsible as I am for this book. I am deeply grateful to have them as friends and mentors.

As early as 1969, Ray Hall, then Safety Officer at the University of Colorado, urged me to write a book on the health and safety hazards involved in art making processes. Ray was among the first to be aware of those dangers and felt that information should be available to everyone working in school environments.

I first proposed to David Baker, editor of *School Arts,* that I write a limited series of health and safety-related articles for the magazine in 1976. His enthusiastic acceptance of that idea led to the "Safetypoint" series, which have been used extensively in writing this book. Dave has been supportive and encouraging, as have all the people at Davis Publications.

Others, too, have made important contributions to this book and if I do not mention all of them, it is only because there are so many. My wife, Betty, has been my constant teacher and critic in the writing of this book. Michael McCann, who reviewed the manuscript, and Monona Rossol have added immeasurably to my understanding of art materials and processes which are inherently hazardous. And over the years many of my students have shared with me their experiences and their attitudes about hazards in the artroom.

Marilyn Newton, Carol Worlock and Karen Greene gave me a number of very helpful insights into how art teachers deal everyday with hazards in their artrooms. Marc Swadener worked with me to devise procedures for the analysis of research data. Comments from readers of my *School Arts* articles have also been very important to me.

CONTENTS

Contents

FOREWORD

Our environment is not particularly benign. Every day newspapers report new potential carcinogens and other dangerous substances in our environment. Accidents regularly claim lives or limbs in homes, schools or workplaces. Few of us are particularly shocked any longer. There seems to be nothing we do that is not in some way harmful. There sometimes seems still less we can do about it.

This book is intended to help art teachers understand the hazards which exist in art processes. It suggests ways to eliminate or deal with them safely. Few claim the artroom can be made completely hazard-free, since we know too well how inventive all of us are in discovering ways to injure ourselves. Nonetheless, teachers can establish procedures in the artroom by which students learn safe and effective ways of doing art activities. Most hazards are unnecessary, and in those processes where hazards are inherent, it is usually possible to minimize them.

Art programs need not be destroyed in the elimination of hazardous art materials or practices. Correcting problems is not always expensive, nor should calling attention to them necessarily threaten an art teacher's program or job. The chapters ahead will identify potential problems and point out solutions. Such an approach will not only reduce the possibility of illness or accidents but may even result in a better overall art program.

Some 100,000 man-made chemicals exist. Some are unquestionably beneficial — we use them to heal the sick, to produce fabrics and to grow food. Many of these chemicals, though, are dangerous and are of real concern to us.

As artists and teachers, we use chemicals every day in the classroom. The hazards of some of them have become a worry. We know of both teachers and students who have had adverse reactions to certain materials. Some have suffered serious illness probably caused by substances used in making art. This new worry augments our old concern about injuries. As art teachers, we wonder if we are doing all we can to spare students and ourselves illness or injury. Consequently, we want to be sure everyone learns safe ways of working in the artroom.

Art should be a joyful experience for both student and teacher. It provides ways for students to experience a richer world. Injury or illness should not be allowed to spoil this experience.

Part 1

OVERVIEW: PROBLEMS AND ANSWERS

1

Artroom Hazards: The Reality

THE NEED FOR ACTION

The artroom more closely resembles an industrial environment than it does a regular classroom. Many are unaware that making art often requires more than an easel, a single brush and pan of watercolor. Of all the different educational settings, the artroom, along with the industrial arts shop and the chemistry lab, relies on specialized equipment, tools and materials. At all grade levels, the artroom should be considered apart from the regular classroom. Whatever the intensity of the program, precautions must be taken to insure that working with art materials does not lead to student illness or injury.

Some art activities are obviously more complex than others and require many more tools and materials. As complexity increases, so do the hazards. If all art were drawing with a #2 pencil or painting with watercolor, there would be few problems to concern teachers. But art education has broadened to include many materials and techniques once thought limited to industrial operations.

Some teachers are aware that health and safety risks exist in their artrooms but choose to do nothing about them. They fear the cost of making corrections will either force the abandonment of parts of their program or give an unsympathetic administrator the chance to eliminate art altogether. That fear may be well founded in some situations. However, a teacher who intentionally takes this course of action invites serious consequences; some risks may well result in student illness or injury and ultimately in the unpleasantness of litigation. (See Chapter Nine for a discussion of teacher liability.) If there is a risk that a program might be cut when requests are made to correct hazards, there is certainly no doubt the program *will* be cut if an administrator finds teachers who knowingly perpetuate unsafe conditions or practices.

Teachers who are uninformed about potential hazards jeopardize both themselves and their students. Each teacher has the responsibility to know his or her own program well enough to understand the hazards and deal effectively with them. With good planning and careful methods of working, the art program should not suffer for making the necessary corrections, and the students will benefit substantially from the entire process. Moreover, since the teacher is in contact with hazards for the longest period of time, the pay-off may actually be a healthier and longer life.

DEFINING HEALTH AND SAFETY

It is a little artificial to separate the health versus safety hazards in the artroom. Each can result in injury, and often actions taken to eliminate one, eliminate the other. For example, removal of sawdust to reduce the safety hazard of falling on slippery floors also reduces the health hazard caused by breathing dust particles. However, it is customary to distinguish between health and safety hazards by the effects each has on the human body. Those resulting in illness are considered health problems, while those causing injury are considered safety related.

ARTROOM CONDITIONS NATIONWIDE

While most art teachers recognize that some hazards exist in their classrooms, they may get little support for correcting them. An uninformed supervisor or financially strapped principal would rather assume any problems are isolated, unconfirmed and only potentially serious. There may even be teachers who share those views.

In 1984, *School Arts* magazine funded a national art hazards survey (Qualley, p. 47, 1984). More than four hundred art teachers responded with information about teaching practices involving potential health and safety problems. Nearly three hundred were teachers in junior or senior high schools. Their responses leave no doubt that the hazards potential is, in fact, the reality (Qualley and Swadener, p. 41, 1985).

Over three-quarters of junior and senior high school teachers use some electric tools (drills, saws, grinders and heating equipment). Large percentages of the teachers have students working with cutting tools such as scissors, razor blades and X-acto knives. Safety reminder signs are in limited use. Competency testing surveys indicate that 43 percent of art teachers evaluate by observation alone; only 18 percent use written tests. Even fewer junior and senior high school art teachers (12 percent) keep any records of student competency test scores on tool use.

Many art teachers are aware that health and safety hazards exist in classrooms where tools and art materials are used, but even there, practices are often not in the best interests either of the students or themselves. Because information about art hazards has been sparse, most teachers continue to work the way they have always worked and use tools and materials that have been stand-bys for many years. There are, indeed, health and safety problems which teachers need to know about and correct if safe working conditions are to exist in the artroom.

For example, consider the survey findings on asbestos glove use. Depending on their construction and condition, they may or may not pose a serious problem. But the well-publicized carcinogenic properties of asbestos should cause teachers to avoid asbestos gloves in general. Yet, 29 percent of high schools and 11 percent of junior highs report their use.

Poor ventilation is one of the most important health problems in schools. It has not been well-solved in most schools. The survey shows that kilns are fired during school hours by a large majority of teachers; nearly half of the firing is done in classrooms with only general ventilation. Since opening windows and doors provides the only ventilation in 88 percent of junior and senior high school artrooms, a large number of students are breathing gases or fumes from kiln firing for several hours each time. The dangers of this depend on what is being fired, but carbon monoxide (from the combustion of organic matter in clay) is produced by all kilns. Sulfur dioxide and nitrogen oxides are often produced. It is also impossible to assess the toxicity of the chemical fumes combined during glaze firing. Few teachers report firing their kilns before or after school hours when fewer people are around, even though many have automatic controls to provide safety backup. Unfortunately, only 18 percent report their kilns are vented through a canopy hood, the most effective type of ventilation.

Solvents are another serious artroom hazard. Fortunately, most teachers (80 percent) store only small quantities and seem to keep them in their original containers, perhaps with the label warnings intact, but few have fireproof cabinets for them. Disposal of waste solvents is also a serious matter. One-quarter of the teachers surveyed dilute solvents with water and put them down the drain. This practice can create serious problems in water purification systems. One-half put solvents in the trash for regular disposal—a fire hazard and a health hazard because of escaping fumes. If solvents are to be used and kept in the room, far more attention needs to be given proper disposal methods.

Airplane glue, rubber cement and wheat paste are very popular at all grade levels, even though their use should be greatly curtailed. Airplane glue is extremely toxic, and rubber cement contains solvents that should not be used with children under twelve. When rubber cement is used in secondary schools, there should always be good ventilation; in 88 percent of the classrooms, ventilation is by opening windows, and that usually is inadequate. Wheat paste (commercial wall paper paste), which contains toxic preservatives, is used in 63 percent of the elementary classrooms and 53 percent of all schools. Teachers should be very careful in the use of all of these adhesives and be sure the ventilation is more than adequate for the material used.

Permanent type markers contain aromatic hydrocarbons and other organic solvents which can be very toxic unless ventilation is extremely good. Even then they should only be used when absolutely necessary. At the elementary level, they should *never* be used. Yet they are used in 70 percent of all classrooms and in 70 percent of junior and senior high art classrooms. Since markers are among the most popular of all art materials, more attention must be given to substituting water-based brands whenever possible.

Few teachers surveyed seem to have noticed the AP (Approved Product) or CP (Certified Product) seals of the Art and Craft Materials Institute which would insure the non-toxicity of their materials. Most (82 percent) have noticed "non-toxic" on labels, but of that number, how many know what this designation really means?

Potential problems are very real given these findings. What emerges is a picture of teachers without an understanding of the dangers of some tools and materials used in the classroom and without any programmatic way of instructing and testing students in the use of those tools and materials.

2

The First Steps: Teacher- Student Cooperation

THE TEACHER'S ROLE

Naturally, the teacher is the single most important factor in providing health and safety instruction and supervision. Without a teacher committed to a health and safety program, even the most complete guidelines will be of little value. Such a program must be specifically designed for the conditions existing in each classroom. Consistent instruction and enforcement of rules will inspire students with the same respect for art hazards.

Prevention is the key: students should avoid materials that may make them sick and techniques that can injure them. With that as a fundamental premise, the following generalizations can form the basis for an effective health and safety program.

First, good classroom management reduces accidents and injuries as well as health problems. Second, less toxic materials can usually be suitably substituted for toxic ones with little or no extra cost. Third, learning how to use tools and equipment correctly and safely is no more difficult than learning to use them incorrectly. And fourth, remember that practices learned in the classroom will be those the students follow elsewhere and in subsequent years.

Setting up a program begins with a thorough understanding of existing conditions; the information must be very specific. To get started, the teacher should list existing conditions, carefully examine current materials and practices and know student ages and health characteristics.

Gathering this information may seem difficult and time-consuming, but it is absolutely necessary for the program to work. The outline of sample questions below highlights the type of information which must be gathered. Later chapters provide specific suggestions for gathering information and using it to make the artroom a safe and healthy environment.

General Classroom Conditions

- Housekeeping: Is there dirt, debris and dust? Is there adequate storage and access? Are there information and warning signs?
- Tools and equipment: What is their placement and condition? Is there a maintenance schedule for them?
- Lighting: Is natural and artificial light adequate?
- Ventilation: What are the provisions for general and local fresh air sources?

Current Practices

- Instructional methods: How and to what extent are health and safety included?
- Students' responsibility: What is expected of them? What is their responsibility based on?
- Monitoring procedures: Who insures that correct practices are followed? What are the effects of infractions?
- Classroom management: How are the distribution and pickup of tools, the handling of hazardous materials and the disposal of hazardous waste handled?

Age and Risk Group

- Bodily development: What are the natural defenses for this age? Is manual dexterity well developed?
- Human weaknesses: Which students may have allergies, chemical sensitivities or respiratory problems?

- Exposure accumulation: What is the frequency and term of exposure? Is a medical record kept for teachers who have long-term exposure?
- Skill development: Do students have adequate knowledge of correct procedures or do they take things for granted?

Materials and Activities

- Toxicity: What are the relative ratings of materials used?
- Ingestion, inhalation and absorption through the skin: What are the possibilities of these occurring?
- Power tools: Is the noise level a problem? Are tools located or used with concern for safety?
- Activities in the curriculum: Have they been selected to minimize problems?

The teacher, being fully familiar with the classroom and curriculum, is the one person who can compile this information, but help can come from the school nurse, the principal, teacher aides, concerned parents and students. Each of these persons has a stake in promoting a safe art environment.

This information itself does not create a health and safety program, but it provides the basis for one. Thus, when a teacher is fully aware of existing conditions, the next step will be to instate appropriate practices. In so doing, a health and safety program is established.

STUDENT AWARENESS

The purpose of hazards instruction in the artroom is not to frighten anyone into feeling that only blunt pencils and plain paper pads are safe to work with. It is to call attention to the fact that art materials and processes, like many other things encountered in daily living, can be harmful if we are careless. An attitude of respect must prevail not only for the art objects themselves but for the way those objects are made and for the materials from which they are made. Being afraid to work with a material or tool makes little sense, and it is a teacher's responsibility to provide instruction that will alleviate, not incite, that fear. The teacher is a role model for the students and, as such, must be especially careful to show respect for art processes and to demonstrate a sure knowledge of how to eliminate potential problems.

Students come to the artroom with no real understanding of the dangers involved with the materials or tools they will use. Even though some will be familiar with the art processes, most students are totally unaware these processes may involve problems that could affect their health or safety. Nor should they be expected to know proper methods for working with tools or handling materials.

Having studied the classroom to determine where potential problems exist, find out what the students understand about those problems. To discover exactly what the students know about a process before they begin it, use a simple pre-activity test. From the results, the teacher can tailor, for a specific group, instruction and expectations.

Give a pre-test for every activity covering what they know about the process, the tools, the techniques and the hazards. Such testing is not a terrific burden and can have an important place in art instruction.

Teachers already use lectures, slides, ditto instructional hand-outs and demonstrations to introduce new activities. Finding out what students already know is another important introduction. Some students may know the process before and find another introduction boring; others may be so uninformed that typical methods of introduction will be totally inadequate.

A short pre-test will provide the following information:

1. Have they done this process before in another school or class?
2. Have they already mastered the skills required?
3. Do they know how to use the necessary tools?
4. Do they understand the possible hazards of the process?
5. Do they have examples of previous work?

What are some specific art hazards questions that might be included in this pre-activity test? Figure 1 is a sample test for a linoleum block printing project and can be used as a model. Completing this test several days ahead of a new activity will enable the teacher to devise the best introduction. It will provide valuable information for health and safety information. Large blocks of class time need not be spent on art hazards

PRE ACTIVITY TEST FOR LINOLEUM BLOCK PRINTING

Student name: _____

Date: _____

Teacher's name: _____

1. What is the purpose of using a bench hook?

2. How can you tell when a cutting tool is dull and should be replaced?

3. What is the reason for avoiding getting oil-based ink on your hands?

4. How should you handle the solvent you use in cleaning the block?

5. Where should you put dirty rags after you have used them for cleaning up?

_____

Answers:

1. A bench hook keeps the block from slipping while it is being cut; it is the correct way to hold a block while cutting; it helps determine the direction cuts should go.

2. A tool is dull when it slips or slides across the block surface; dull tools slip and cause injury.

3. To keep the skin from having direct contact with solvents necessary to remove the ink; solvents can cause skin irritation or other problems.

4. Be sure to wear protective gloves; use the smallest amount of solvent possible to do the job; be sure the cleaning is done in a well-ventilated place or in the place the teacher indicates.

5. Solvent-soaked rags are very flammable and special self-closing cans should be used for disposal; fumes from dirty rags can be dangerous to breathe. Rags with solvent in them which need to be saved should be hung under an operating canopy ventilating hood to insure the fumes are drawn out of the room.

Figure 1.

instruction if students already have a good understanding of the correct ways of using the materials and tools required for a planned activity.

Paperwork is already a big problem in schools. Teachers are expected to keep many records. But in this case the extra paperwork helps identify student understanding of a process and is worth the effort.

When students do not do well with the answers to these questions, special emphasis on hazards should be included in the general introduction-demonstration for the project. However, if they do know the answers, only general reminders along with any special information unique to conditions in the present classroom will be necessary. Should it ever be needed, this written test will also serve as evidence that the students demonstrated they knew how to deal with the hazards of the activity.

Daily lesson plans should always include health and safety notes. These notes need not be extensive but will remind teachers of things the students should know about the materials they are using (e.g., "remind the class not to spray fixative inside the classroom"). Awareness of hazards concerns will become second nature both to students and teacher if discussed on a regular basis. Lesson plan formats are usually either prescribed by the individual school or are a very personal design of the teacher. Whichever is the case, planning for health and safety should be "built into" the form used. Consider the format in Figure 2 as one way of doing this.

STUDENT COMMITTEES

Most teachers know that the more students are involved in planning and carrying out learning activities, the more effective learning will be. This holds true for all subjects at any grade level — health and safety instruction is no exception. Enlisting direct student participation produces positive results.

A health and safety committee for the school is one way to do this, but forming such a committee in each class is better yet. What does such a committee do? Its members can work with the teacher in identifying artroom hazards and help design ways to instruct other students in dealing with those problems. They may also make inventories of the materials in the classroom, check label information about toxicity, discover which materials need special storage considerations and establish procedures to guarantee that safe practices are followed.

SAMPLE LESSON PLAN

*Grade: _____ Teacher: _____ Date: _____
*Activity: _____ Planned
Length: _____

Objectives:		
Supplies and Equipment	Have Order	Safety and Health Hazards
Motivation:		
Procedures (continue on back):		
Evaluation:		

Figure 2.

What these committees accomplish obviously depends on the age and maturity of the students, but beginning in the primary grades, children can either volunteer or be selected to meet and talk about health and safety hazards. Perhaps the discussion with young children would involve only scissors safety, but with older students more complex issues can be discussed:

- What does the word toxic mean?
- How can we find out about the toxicity of materials?
- What do we do with materials when we don't know if they are toxic or not?
- Should we make rules about working with art materials?
- How will we know the rules are being followed?
- What will the penalties be for not following the rules?
- How can we make health and safety rules known to the rest of the class?

Students and teacher can decide what materials or practices should be limited or not allowed. Students can help devise ways to monitor and enforce rules and can also work with the school administration in solving critical problems.

Encourage your students to shoulder some of the work involved in health and safety education. Have them involve other students in an important aspect of curriculum planning which will increase learning all around. They will also be useful in suggesting to the school administration changes or improvements in how materials are purchased or in the physical conditions in the classrooms. Involving the students in this way also demonstrates that the teacher is fulfilling a significant responsibility in the health and safety aspects of art education.

Obviously, health and safety education cannot be left entirely to student committees, but the program effectiveness will be enhanced by actively involving students in the process.

3

Precaution
and Protection

BASIC HAZARDS ELIMINATION

The best way to eliminate a hazard is to eliminate its cause. Evaluate any hazardous activity or material in use and determine if its educational value is worth the time, money and effort necessary to overcome the problem it creates. The philosophy of this book is to emphasize several fairly simple methods for reducing artroom health and safety hazards. These suggestions are based on good sense, good housekeeping and the importance of eliminating as many activities involving hazards as is consistent with good art education. Keeping the artroom clean and orderly is one effective means of controlling hazards. Teaching all students to be responsible in their handling and use of materials and tools is yet another important aspect of safe art-making.

Few students respond well to nagging, but reminders must be constantly visible and signs are a useful device for this purpose. And because accidents sometimes do occur, there must be a plan to deal with injury. The teacher should also understand overall first aid requirements for the classroom. These various elements are all important in eliminating hazards and must be a part of a health and safety program.

NO-COST IMPROVEMENTS

Before a good case can be made for spending any funds to reduce hazards, teachers must achieve all that can be done without cost. Clean the artroom;

put supply cabinets in order and label all supplies; reorganize activities to limit or confine problems; and get rid of unusable materials. An objective appraisal will identify much that is cluttering artroom space, creating dust and difficult working conditions.

When these first steps have been taken, it will be easier to enlist the cooperation of others. The inertia will have been broken. Few teachers enjoy artroom housekeeping, but a positive attitude toward it is necessary if health and safety hazards are to be controlled.

Clay, plaster, fiber and everyday dust are usually serious artroom problems; reorganize work procedures so that unavoidable dust is not unnecessarily stirred up. Confine activities like clay mixing to a separate room limited to times when few students are around. These actions cost no money but make obvious and important contributions to hazards elimination. Other points:

- Is the disposal of waste material done properly?
- Are tools carefully stored?
- Are there room and materials inventories?
- Have you developed a set of records showing the scope of your health and safety actions?

These no-cost improvements will indicate to administrators a serious intent to correct hazards. It is the most effective step toward getting financial support to solve the remaining problems.

SIGNS

Signs are no substitute for a teacher's instructional responsibilities or student knowledge. But the selective use, proper placement and periodic changing of signs can effectively remind students of hazards without resorting to nagging.

Any sign is only as effective as its placement and the clarity and pertinence of its message. Obviously, a sign must be displayed where it can be seen and the message must be quickly understood. Signs must be selective—analyze the routine activities of the art program and establish a priority for signs. What are the signs for: to warn, instruct or remind? A sign displayed on or near the paper cutter may be used either to warn of its hazards or remind the student how to use it. "Danger: Watch your fingers!" might be alternated every three or four weeks with "Sharp blade. Keep fingers well back." Changing signs and their location reduces the problem of familiarity resulting in the message being overlooked. Signs that never change are often not seen and have little or no impact on student actions.

What sort of signs should be used? How many should there be? How often should they be changed? Each classroom is different, so each teacher must decide what will probably work best. Some suggestions that will provide guidance are found in Figure 3.

CLOTHING

Many schools have dress codes. Whatever one's attitude is toward these regulations, the art teacher should establish a code applying specifically to dress in the artroom. Such a code has far less to do with style than safety, nothing to do with propriety but much to do with protection. These regulations should also apply to hair and jewelry, since these also represent potential problems in working with tools and equipment.

Students may often not be aware of what can happen when long hair becomes entangled on the spindle of the bench grinder or a loose sleeve or dangling bracelet is wrapped around the bit of a drill press. No one enjoys horror stories about students being scalped or mangled, but such things have happened.

Simple and well enforced rules about clothing, jewelry and hair are appropriate for the artroom. It is, after all, a work area and not a center for fashion display. There should be few objections from any but the most frivolous students. To establish an artroom code, work with the students to identify hazards and develop rules to overcome them. Involving the students in this process usually makes rules more palatable to them. A precedent of past injuries need not exist to justify preventive measures—the purpose is always to prevent accidents, not prove they can happen. With hazards identified and a code designed, a meeting with the principal can establish enforcement methods and clarify the role of the administration.

Once established, the code must be taken seriously. If hair must be tied back, see that it is; if loose clothing is not allowed, require the

USING SIGNS IN THE ARTROOM

Sign Message	Suggested Placement	Frequency of Change
Eye Protection; Safety glasses (WEAR YOUR SAFETY GLASSES)	Above benches in the area where they are to be used.	Rotate position every month or six weeks.
Fire extinguisher location (FIRE EXTINGUISHER IS NEAR THE DOOR)	Near doors or flammable materials; close to extinguisher.	Change design twice a year.
Proper handling and storage of flammable materials. (KEEP CON-TAINERS COVERED)	Inside the storage area.	Change signs two or three times a year.
First aid equipment location. (FIRST AID STATION)	Close to materials	At the beginning of each semester.
Exhaust hood fan (TURN ON FAN)	On hood itself; at eye level.	Change design each semester.
Handling restrictions on equipment. (USE ONLY AFTER INSTRUCTION)	At equipment site; on large equipment.	Each semester.

Figure 3.

student to change or leave the working area; if bracelets or necklaces must be removed, be sure they are. There should be no exceptions, including the teacher.

Accidents sometimes occur in any setting, but there is never a reason for hair, loose clothing or dangling jewelry to cause them. A well thought-out artroom dress code should help see that they don't.

PROTECTIVE EQUIPMENT

The need for individual protective equipment such as safety glasses, respirators or gloves should never exist in the elementary art program because materials requiring them should not be used at that level. Perhaps at the junior high level, some personal protective equipment may be necessary when working with ceramics or jewelry. But it is in the senior high where many activities produce dust or fumes or require contact with hot or sharp materials. Serious consideration must be given to this type equipment.

Personal protective equipment shields the individual from direct exposure to unavoidable dust, mist, vapors, flying particles, chemicals and noise. Generally, much of this equipment should be considered a "last resort" and used only when all other measures have proven inadequate. Good housekeeping, adequate ventilation and substitution of materials must first be fully implemented, because they are fundamentally better techniques. Most personal protective devices are clumsy, uncomfortable and expensive. Often they create problems, because students do not want to use them regularly, do not adapt to them well and either actively resist using them or simply "forget." Sometimes using such equipment cannot be avoided, but it should never be considered a panacea for artroom hazards or a quick-fix for environmental problems.

Eye protection is necessary in the grinding and polishing of jewelry, chipping and carving of sculptured forms and cutting and sanding of wood. Wearing safety goggles is in fact required by law, and students usually do so in obvious situations because this form of protective equipment has become fairly standard. Only two points need to be made: be sure they are used and be sure to select the correct goggles for the job. They should be flexible-fitting, have regular ventilation built in and have a wide angle of vision. However, the so-called eye-cup type may be needed for certain welding and chipping activities because they fit closely to the face. Be sure the goggles fit properly, and give special attention to students who wear eye glasses or contact lenses. Where chemical fumes are involved, students wearing contact lenses should not wear ventilated goggles, since vapors or gases can become concentrated under or absorbed by the lenses and cause serious eye irritation. Safety goggles are easily scratched and vision can be significantly impaired, so they must be replaced when this occurs. Elastic head bands eventually stretch and become loose so they should frequently be replaced as well.

Respirators and masks filter out harmful vapors and dust, but the correct NIOSH-approved filter must be used or the expected protection may be missing. (NIOSH refers to the National Institute for Occupational Safety and Health.) The fit is critical, since a mask or respirator which allows dust, vapors or other airborne material to enter around the edges has no value. Product information should be read carefully before ordering to be certain the filter selected will remove the type of dust or vapors that represent the hazard. These will probably be materials such as the free silica in clay powder or organic vapors from solvents and lacquer thinners. Do not expect that masks will filter out gases and fumes from kiln firing since too many different fumes are produced for any one mask to be effective.

   Respirator use must be carefully limited because most of them make breathing difficult. Students with any respiratory or heart problems should use them only with their doctor's approval. Perhaps more than any other personal protective equipment, respirators should be used only under extreme situations: when local exhaust ventilation is impractical for some very limited or infrequently done operation or while a regular ventilation system is temporarily out of order. Although beards are seldom found on students in schools, teachers should, for their own benefit, be aware that a beard prevents a proper fit around a respirator and completely negates any protection it might be thought to offer.

Gloves are available in a variety of materials, designed to protect against specific chemical damage. In normal artroom activities, disposable vinyl or polyethylene gloves are usually adequate. These are thin enough to provide the tactile sensitivity necessary for most activities, are resistant to limited exposures of most chemicals and are relatively inexpensive. For the limited amount of solvents used in most artrooms, these will provide the protection if they are replaced as soon as they give any evidence of wear or leakage. Be sure they are long enough to cover the wrists.

Protective skin creams, or "barrier creams," are also available in cases where gloves cannot be used. They must be re-applied after any hand washing and must also be renewed frequently if they are to be effective. For both gloves and barrier creams, know the specific chemicals being handled and check manufacturer's information concerning the best glove material to use for the expected protection. Some gloves are very expensive, so be sure they will do the job.

Noise from machine use will not be frequent or consistent enough to require ear protection in most art classrooms, but noise problems should not be overlooked. Grinders, buffers, saws and sanders may require students to wear ear plugs or sound insulated ear covers. First reduce machine noise through proper mounting and maintenance. Install sound absorbing materials around the machine area, and limit the time any individual or class is exposed to the noise. Ear protectors should be available near any noisy machine so students can use them when they feel a need. But in most artrooms, their use need not be mandatory.

Personal protective equipment should certainly be used in some regular art activities: NIOSH-approved dust masks for the mixing of clay or powdered dyes and pigments; gloves for working with oil-based printing inks and any solvents; and safety glasses for grinding or chipping various materials. Any other protective equipment should be used only when there is no other option. When it must be used, the fit must be perfect. Select this equipment carefully to protect against specific hazards, or it can be a waste of time and money.

FIRST AID

In most schools, a nurse is usually on duty at least part of the time. Art teachers often develop a false sense of security with that knowledge. When possible, sending the student to the nurse is the wisest action, but there may be times when this cannot be done. The nurse may not be in the building or the injury may be too severe and require instant attention. The teacher must know immediately what to do.

Long before the need arises, the art teacher should meet with the school nurse (or district nurse if the individual school does not have one) and get information and/or instruction on first aid. A first aid kit containing antiseptics, bandages and compresses should be prepared for the room, and the teacher's instruction should include when and how to use them. Ideally, all art teachers in the district should have a session during which they receive help and have the opportunity to practice techniques of immediate treatment. Apart from general first aid, teachers should be taught to respond to the specific types of injury or illness that may actually occur in the artroom: wounds, burns, shock or the ingestion of poisons. Knowing CPR techniques may be extremely useful in everyday life, but it is far less likely to be needed in the classroom than knowing how to deal with severe bleeding or a second degree burn.

Wounds and Bleeding

- Don't dismiss slight wounds and scratches. They should be washed thoroughly and covered with a sterile dressing.
- Encourage puncture wounds to bleed a little to flush out foreign material. Any wound has the potential for developing tetanus and should be treated accordingly.
- Apply a sterile dressing to prevent entrance of additional germs.
- Wash hands with soap and water to reduce contamination of the dressing as it is applied.
- Stop severe bleeding with a clean cloth pad (preferably sterile) pressed against the wound. If the bleeding continues, add another pad and hold tightly on top of the first. Have the student lie down and, if the wound is on an arm or leg, elevate it. Immediately send for help.

Burns

- First degree burns redden the surface of the skin. Cool the site with cold water and cover with a sterile dressing. Physicians often discourage the immediate application of burn ointments because the

person may be sensitive to them and they may be difficult to remove later.
- Second degree burns cause blisters. Cool with cold water and carefully cover with a sterile dressing without breaking the blister.
- Third degree burns destroy the underlying growth cells. Treat as other burns, if possible. For extensive burns, don't attempt to remove clothing. Treat for shock.
- Get the student to help as quickly as possible for second and third degree burns, especially if they cover a significant area.
- Flush chemical burns with large quantities of water; continue flushing until help arrives.

Shock

- Shock is caused by a failure of the circulatory system and occurs after burns, emotional stress or loss of blood.
- Make the injured person lie down, with head low to maintain blood supply to the brain; keep him or her comfortably warm, but cover only if chilly.
- Call for medical assistance immediately.

Poisoning by Mouth

- Give water or milk in large quantities; include Ipecac syrup in first aid kits to induce vomiting.
- Find the poison container and look for antidote instructions: follow them carefully and call a physician or poison control center immediately.
- Do not induce vomiting if the poisoning is from kerosene or other petroleum products or from any caustics such as acid.

The preceding is intended only to give some general insight into first aid for the artroom. It should not be considered adequate instruction in proper first aid treatment. These injuries are not the only kinds possible in the artroom. There is a great need for first aid information, and teachers are well advised to get assistance from the school medical personnel before it is required.

VENTILATION

Ventilation is the key to solving many of the most serious health hazards in the artroom. The warning found on labels to "use with adequate ventilation" calls attention to the problem but provides no understanding of what is adequate. Ventilation requirements differ according to the setting: size of the room, numbers and ages of the students and the concentration of hazardous fumes.

With effective and complete ventilation, there is almost no art material which cannot be used safely (Carnow, 1981). However, no classroom will automatically have perfect ventilation for every substance, and teachers must know what contaminants must be removed and what systems are necessary to do the job. Simply opening a window will not be sufficient.

In making plans for proper ventilation, start with the information gathered in a materials inventory. Try several sources for ventilation advice: the science department in one of your schools may have information or the local department of public or environmental health, for example. But it is not easy or inexpensive to find people with expertise in designing artroom ventilation systems. Even the most highly qualified industrial ventilation specialists will need specific information about the kind and amount of contaminants before they can make judgments. The *Accident Prevention Manual for Industrial Operations* (McElroy, 1969) is thorough and clear but does not deal with school settings as such, and the information must be extrapolated. An excellent source of ventilation information is *Ventilation A Practical Guide* (Clark, et al, 1984) which is written for application to artists' studios and comes closest to addressing the needs of the art classroom. The ventilation requirements for many materials are complex, and the best and most practical approach is to eliminate problem materials.

When as many of these materials have been eliminated as is possible, determine if the general (room-wide) ventilation is sufficient or whether the activities which require materials that produce fumes or dust can be concentrated in a smaller space. If they can be confined, a local exhaust system, such as a vent with fan, should be able to remove the contaminants before they disburse throughout the entire room. It is far easier to ventilate a small space than a large one. An example of this would be the fumes from melting wax for batik, which should be drawn completely away from the space where people are working with the materials and should not be allowed to spread through the classroom. Several possible ventilation methods are shown in Figure 4.

Consider electric kilns: many are located inside the artroom so that a canopy hood is necessary to remove the fumes generated. Kiln fumes are a special problem because they are released by a variety of substances in the firing process, and their exact nature is not often known. It might be possible to fire a kiln without a ventilating hood if it were done at night when the room and building are empty, but unattended firing is extremely hazardous and may well result in serious damage to the kiln or to the building itself. So long as people remain in the building, they may well be in some danger from the fumes. There is also a possibility that fumes may linger and still be present in the building the next morning. Excellent and clear suggestions for electric kiln ventilation design that can be directly applied to the art room are provided by Clark, Cutter and McGrane (pp. 69-71).

Before those expensive solutions are undertaken, eliminate problem materials through substitution, and confine activities which generate fumes, gases, or dust to places where contamination is most easily extracted. Keep the room clean. Be guided in your planning by the following "Rules for Good Ventilation" (Clark, et al, pp. 22-23):

1. Direct air flow away from breathing zones of people who work in the area.
2. Exhaust contaminated air from the workspace.
3. Place the exhaust opening of the ventilation system as close as possible to the source of the contaminants.
4. Avoid crossdrafts.
5. Supply make-up air to replace the air exhausted by the ventilation system.
6. Discharge the contaminated air away from openings that draw air into the studio or shop.
7. Avoid polluting the community.

Ventilation systems produce heat loss in cold weather climates, because air replacing the exhausted air usually comes from the outside. How much does this amount to in added heating costs? To estimate this figure

POSSIBLE VENTILATION DESIGNS

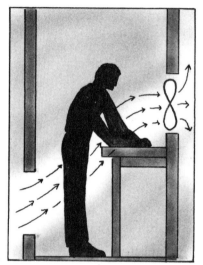

General purpose ventilation with fan to outside.

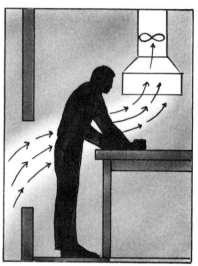

Canopy hood for print inking, acid etching, ceramic kilns, foundries.

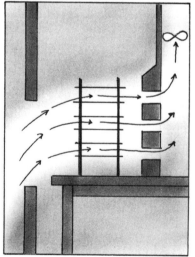

Slotted hood for drying prints, silk screen printing, soldering.

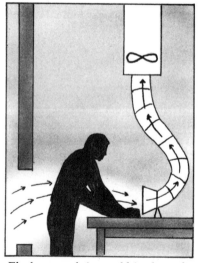

Elephant trunk (moveable) exhaust for welding, woodworking machines.

Figure 4.

for a specific location, a ventilation engineer can calculate hourly and yearly costs of tempering (heating up) the air by using equations designed for that purpose (Loeffler, pp. 7–11).

To minimize this cost, system designers usually will try to use one of the following methods of conservation:

- Reduction in the volume of air handled. This may be done by reducing hours of use, using low-volume high velocity hoods or using other principles of local exhaust capture.
- Delivery of untempered air. Using supply air that has not been preheated may be a way of reducing cost if that air is likely to undergo some heating in the room itself. If, for example, the ventilation system is running only when classes are in session, body heat may be sufficient to keep the room comfortably warm.
- Recovery of energy from exhausted air. Heat exchangers can be used to extract heat from outgoing air. This is usually prohibitive in a classroom setting because of equipment cost.
- Recovery of uncontaminated air. Such a procedure requires primary and secondary air cleaning equipment with automatic monitoring to insure the recirculated air is clean. The cost and complexity of such a system rules it out for the artroom application (Loeffler, pp. 7–15).

A combination of the first and second methods is the most applicable to artroom ventilation requirements. Some heat loss will occur, but that loss must be balanced against the health hazards involved. With careful operation of the ventilation system, energy loss can be kept minimal, and students can be both safe and comfortable.

4

Controlling Artroom Hazards

The artroom is a setting with unique problems resulting from the tools and materials used and the variety of processes performed. What is so unique about the artroom and what health or safety hazards do they create? How can a teacher control the hazards of some of this material so they can be used safely?

FIXED EQUIPMENT LOCATION

Most teachers have learned that the distribution of supplies and equipment affects the success of an art lesson. Equipment also piques the curiosity of many students. If students are to be discouraged from exploring it and risking unnecessary injury, fixed equipment in particular must be placed so that the artroom doesn't become an "attractive nuisance."

Each classroom has different kinds of fixed equipment. Some, such as the electric kiln, are literally wired into one location and can't be moved. Others, like the paper cutter, drying racks and free standing tools, can be moved but seldom are. Teachers must decide where tools will be safest, and when the arrangement has been tested for workability, the equipment should be left permanently in those places. Although there is no one proper configuration for placing equipment, here are some useful guidelines.

Electric kiln location is usually determined by its wiring, venting and by normal room traffic patterns. Fumes from firing must not, of course, be allowed to spread throughout the room and adjoining halls, so a canopy ventilating hood is a requirement. Kiln venting is the major factor in locating the kiln. But it must also be placed away from usual traffic lanes and be separated from the students. Ideally, the kiln should not be located in the classroom itself, but perhaps in an alcove or storage area. If it must be in the classroom, a chain link barrier will keep students away from the kiln when it is hot and at the same time allow the teacher to monitor it visually.

Paper cutters are usually portable and moving them is often a way to clear a table top for other uses. This is a poor practice. If the cutter does not have its own stand, select a table (perhaps one discarded from some other use), shorten the legs so it is the proper height for the students to use, and attach the cutter to it. Put the cutter in an easily observable area of the room so that those who are permitted to use it can be seen.

Saws, drill presses, and other free standing equipment are not uncommon in artrooms. These should be placed in little used areas of the room to insure a clear working space for cutting and drilling. Mark the floor around the machine with wide colored tape or painted strips to show the operator and helper where to stand and to indicate a limit behind which all others must stay. A table saw (rare in an artroom) must have a "safety zone" large enough to protect students from the occasional kick-back of wood improperly fed into the saw. It must be placed in a way that the direction of the blade rotation is away from the class. With proper instruction and supervision, these tools should pose no great safety problems.

Printing presses probably will have to be moved out of the way when not in use, unless the room is used exclusively for printmaking. Attach the press permanently to a table of appropriate size and height. When it is being stored either move it entirely out of the artroom or into an area where it will not interfere with student movement. A press not in use should be covered to protect it from dust, from being used as a storage surface and, most importantly, to discourage students from playing with it. If possible, remove the spokes or drive wheel so that the rollers cannot be turned and so that no one will inadvertently bump into these spokes.

Drying racks should be located where there is good access and the shelves can easily be reached. There is little hazard with such racks except when they are improperly used for general storage — a function for which they were not designed and which may cause them to collapse or to become bent and not work properly. These racks can be used to help define room areas and should be located close to where they are used. Drying racks for silk screen activities using oil-based inks should be vented to carry off the vapors from the evaporating solvents in the ink.

Properly located equipment can make the artroom a safer and more functional place to work. A clear understanding of how the equipment works and the amount of space each piece requires is needed to determine its location. How often and by whom it is used is the second factor in deciding location. This should not be done casually, and once placement is made, it should be tried and changed if it does not work well. When a good location is found, equipment should remain there.

SOLVENTS

If solvents are strong enough to dilute or dissolve oil-based inks and paint or lacquers, it doesn't take much imagination to realize what they can do to human beings. Turpentine and lacquer thinner have been in general artroom use for so long they are often accepted as normal part of everyday life. Yet these and other solvents should not be taken for granted and the hazards they impose must not be overlooked.

As with other substances, the most effective precaution with solvents is to be sure they are necessary. Eliminate the hazard by eliminating its cause.

With the development of high quality and versatile water-based inks and paint, the necessity for solvents other than water has been significantly reduced. Experimentation with acrylic paint should convince students that it is as much an "artist's medium" as is oil paint, and it can be used for any visual effect the student wants. The pigments in some paints may be hazardous, but if students keep it (and their brushes) away from their mouths, the risks are minimal. Water-based silk screen printing materials are very effective and eliminate the need for the extremely toxic solvents normally used in this process. Visual results with these materials may differ somewhat from those with petroleum-based inks, and on very large prints paper shrinkage may cause registration problems. Nevertheless, they provide a genuine experience in all of the screen printing process.

Permanent type materials which require solvents should only be used in properly ventilated rooms, and not at the elementary level. Do not use paint stripper or varnish remover in the artroom under any circumstances. They are probably the most dangerous of solvents and completely unnecessary in any program. Further, be extremely careful to use lacquer thinner only when absolutely necessary, for it too has very toxic contents.

The table in Figure 5 provides information describing the solvents most often found in the artroom. These are reasonably safe if precautions are taken in their use, but there should be very little reason to need them. Not to have them available would be the best overall decision.

STORING DANGEROUS LIQUIDS

Solvents are almost always highly flammable. If they must be used, their handling and storage must be designed to reduce the possibility of fire. A few facts are helpful in doing this. Liquids are considered flammable if they have a flash point below 100° F. They are combustible if their flash point is 100°–140° F. Flash point temperatures listed for substances may vary slightly depending on the evaluating agency making these classifications (McCann, 1979, pp. 67–68). But since the variance is only about 20°, it is simpler to use 100° as the figure differentiating combustible and flammable materials. Flash point is defined as the temperature at which the liquid gives off enough vapor to form a mixture with air near the liquid's surface that will ignite when a flame or spark is present (McElroy, 1969, p. 1010). The lower the flash point, the more flammable the liquid. Flash point is not the temperature at which the material would spontaneously burst into flame, as is sometimes thought.

Flammable liquids (Class I) which might be found in the artroom are acetone, benzene, ethyl alcohol, toluol (contained in some lacquer thinners) and turpentine. Gasoline is also a Class I liquid. None of these are essential for artroom activities. They should not be used or stored in an artroom for any reason, because of their high volatility (the tendency to vaporize or evaporate rapidly), and for the health hazards they create.

SOLVENTS OFTEN FOUND IN THE ARTROOM

Solvent	Hazard	Precautions
Paint Thinner (Petroleum distillates)	Inhalation may cause dizziness; irritating to eyes, nose, throat; causes dry, cracked skin. Affects mostly skin, eyes, respiratory and central nervous systems. Combustible.	Use sparingly; wash after use; keep container closed when not in use. Exercise care against indirect ingestion. Store in a proper cabinet. Do not use in elementary grades.
Turpentine	Irritates eyes, nose, throat and skin. Contact can cause sensitization (subsequent allergenic reaction). Kidney damage. Flammable.	Avoid use. Substitute paint thinner.
Lacquer Thinner (Toluene, Ketones)	Causes dizziness, weakness, muscle fatigue, dermatitis. Inhaling large quantities can cause death. Attacks central nervous system, liver, kidneys, and skin. Flammable.	Limit use to specifically ventilated areas. Keep containers covered when not in use. Store properly. Do not use in elementary grades.
Shellac Thinner (Denatured alcohol)	Poisonous. Irritating to eyes, nose, throat and it is mildly narcotic in small amounts. Flammable.	Should not contain methyl alcohol. Use with close supervision but avoid use if possible. Keep container closed when not in use. Store properly. Do not use in elementary grades.

Figure 5.

Combustible liquids (Class II), such as kerosene, mineral spirits, or lithotine, may be found in some artrooms. These are not as hazardous as Class I materials but still should be stored in special containers and only used when absolutely necessary.

Storage containers used for flammable and combustible liquids should be designed specifically for them. The best container will be of heavy metal with a spring-closing lid. Figure 6 outlines maximum quantities of these liquids that can be stored in several types of containers.

Storage cabinets for flammable and combustible liquids should be double-walled, built of 18 gauge metal and have tightly closing, lockable doors. One inch thick plywood with glued and screwed joints can be substituted, but doors should fit tightly and hinges should be sturdy enough to keep the doors from sagging. These cabinets are intended to keep fire from reaching their contents and should meet the NFPA (National Fire Protection Association) fire code. If that is not possible, have any cabinet used for this purpose approved by the local fire marshal. Clearly label the cabinet "Flammable—Keep Fire Away." Open containers should never be left in any storage cabinet.

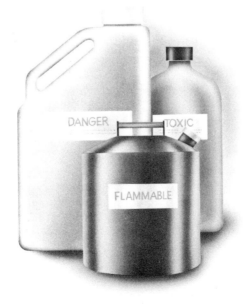

STORAGE CONTAINERS
FOR FLAMMABLE AND COMBUSTIBLE LIQUIDS

	Class IC* Flammable	Class II Combustible
Glass or plastic**	up to 1 gallon	1 gallon
Metal	1 to 2 gallons	1 gallon
Safety cans	2 gallons	2 gallons

*Class IA and IB flammable liquids should not normally be kept in an artroom since there would be no reasonable use for them. (Among them are ethyl ether, acetone, benzol, benzine, ethyl acetate, ethyl alcohol, gasoline, methanol and methyl ethyl ketone.) Only flammable aerosol sprays (a Class IA substance) might be used in an artroom.

**Always use non-breakable containers if possible. All must be labeled to identify their contents clearly. Keep containers covered except when actually in use to reduce the vapors in the air around the work area.

Figure 6.

Waste disposal of rags or paper towels that have been used with flammable or combustible liquids should be in an approved waste container. These cans are constructed of sheet metal and have covers designed to open only partially. When released, covers will close automatically. These containers must be emptied at the end of every school day. The disposal of any waste or any waste solvents must be handled differently from normal trash.

Disposal of solvent-contaminated waste will vary from school to school. It is the teacher's responsibility to alert both the principal and custodian to the fact that there is such waste and that it should be handled according to school district or local government policies. Make this notification in writing, indicating how much waste is likely to exist and how often it will need to be emptied.

Self-closing containers, approved cabinets and acceptable waste containers are necessary if any combustible liquids are used. This equipment will significantly reduce the possibility of fire. However, real fire safety depends on consistent monitoring to be sure that proper procedures are followed. Always be sure nothing is kept in the artroom that is not necessary.

ADHESIVES

Scissors, paste and colored crayons: there probably isn't a classroom in the country where they won't be found, even in places where there is no art program as such. They rank as the most basic materials in art education. Of the three, paste is worth particular attention because it is so often taken for granted. Paste — or the more generic term, adhesive — comes in many different forms and has many different purposes. So there are special problems in its selection and in supervising how it can be used safely in the classroom.

School paste is the most commonly used general purpose paste. It is thick and difficult to spread except with fingers (which often get "cleaned off" in the mouth — even by older students). It works reasonably well in fastening paper to paper but cracks and dries out, so it is not usually very permanent. School paste is not especially effective in fastening cloth to cloth or to paper and does not hold wood or toothpick constructions together. This type of paste smells inviting to students and some may intentionally eat it, but non-toxic brands can be found and it is generally safe for classroom use.

White glue is probably the most popular glue used in or out of the school because of its versatility and strength. It dries transparently and permanently. It can also be thinned with water for gluing paper to paper and is thus especially economical. Its smell and taste are not particularly inviting and most brands are non-toxic, generally safe for classroom use.

Rubber cement adheres paper to paper quickly, though not permanently, cleans off easily when dry (except from clothing) but does stain colored paper. It is highly flammable and contains volatile (fast evaporating) solvents such as hexane and other aromatic hydrocarbons which are extremely hazardous when inhaled. Hexane, for example, has sometimes been known to cause dizziness, numbness and even paralysis. Aerosol (spray) cements are similar in composition to rubber cement and create more problems because the particles are forcefully airborne.

Do not use rubber cement with children under twelve. When used by older students, keep the jars tightly closed except when the brush is actually in use so the fumes are contained as much as possible. Work only in a very well ventilated space. Keep in mind that open windows are only effective for ventilation if there is enough air coming in to make up for the air going out (cross ventilation), and remember that it is likely that windows will be open only when the weather is warm. Planning art activities to coincide with nice weather conditions is not the way to have a particularly predictable program.

Non-flammable rubber cement is now available. However, until its chemical composition is known for sure, it should be assumed that it may contain 1,1,1-trichloroethane (methyl chloroform) which is toxic. Thus, while the problem of flammability may have been solved, use rubber cement only when absolutely necessary and then with excellent ventilation.

Wheat paste (wallpaper paste) comes in powder form and is mixed with water for use. It is an excellent, inexpensive paste, often used for papier-mâché, but the specific kind used must be selected carefully. Wheat paste is made to stick wallpaper to walls and most of it is toxic; it contains rodent poison and sometimes toxic mercury preservatives. Using only those brands identified as non-toxic may reduce concern, but this may be misleading. If there is nothing on the label about toxicity, do not use it at all. You must assume some of it will wind up in the students' mouths.

Airplane glue (model cement) is expensive and of limited usefulness except in lightweight, three-dimensional constructions. It is extremely flammable and contains toluene which is highly toxic if inhaled; it should not be used in the elementary grades. Use with other students should be strictly limited and carefully monitored.

Glue sticks are handy and easy to use, relatively inexpensive, work well for most paper to paper gluing and are usually non-toxic.

Avoid any adhesive product that does not provide information as to its contents or warnings about its possible flammability or toxicity.

MAKING A MATERIALS INVENTORY

Controlling potentially hazardous materials is, of course, a primary goal in the artroom. One of the most effective controls is to keep a complete inventory of all art materials used. An inventory provides a record of consumption in order to know how much should be stored in the artroom and to what extent those materials represent a hazard. Any label information gathered in this process can be used to set up materials categories. Label information divides materials into three such categories: non-toxic materials, materials which are harmful under some circumstances and materials whose contents are unknown. Use an inventory sheet, like or similar to that shown in Figure 7 to record:

- Kind of material in the room.
- Number or amount on hand.
- How often each is used.
- Where and how it is stored.
- Who has specific responsibility for it.
- What kind of disposal procedures are required.

This inventory provides a concise record of any materials that may cause health problems as well as immediate information about the amount of all supplies on hand. If current, this inventory will be an excellent way to know the overall status of supplies and expedite ordering any materials. Its primary function, however, is to control hazardous substances. Making this inventory should be an annual activity. And looking for information about toxicity should be a standard part of this inventory process.

SCRAP MATERIALS

Art teachers have been brought up on a regular program of improvisation in their use of materials. Art from throw-aways has historically been the way to extend meager budgets. The practice is considered educationally sound based on the creativity it takes to change trash into objects of beauty. Sometimes it seems almost preferable to use junk in place of new materials. Contemporary interest in recycling even gives the process an environmentally positive twist. With such attitudes, there are probably few art teachers

MATERIALS INVENTORY

TOXIC CONTENT CODE

Non-toxic	A
Toxic	B
Unknown	C

Room Number: _____

Teacher: _____

Date: _____

Quantity	Item	Description	Toxic Code	Notes/Date and amount of re-order

Figure 7

who give more than a passing thought to the boxes and piles of "stuff" they have accumulated. But scrap is as much a part of the regular inventory as are the fresh tempera paint and drawing paper.

Much of what teachers accumulate in the way of "supplementary" supplies is both useful and visually exciting. Wallpaper samples, corrugated cardboard, styrofoam meat trays, scraps of cloth, yarn, wood, buttons, light bulbs, applicator sticks, shoe polish, feathers, bottle caps, mailing tubes, game parts—the list is long. The only limits seem to be the imagination and energy of the teacher and the availability of storage space.

In most cases these materials do not represent any unique health hazard or involve safety risks that are not obvious. The greatest problem is that their composition is unknown. If wood scraps are painted, what is the content of the paint? Was toxic dye used to color the feathers? Did the applicator sticks come fresh from a package or were they used for some unknown purpose before they got to the artroom? Who can guess what is in shoe polish except various kinds of waxes, and what is known about them? In general, there is no way to find out about any scrap materials. There is little possibility of tracing the materials, and it is unlikely there will be information on any label. Not knowing, then, means taking special care in their use:

- Wash hands frequently.
- Keep storage containers clean and free of dust.
- Keep all materials out of the mouth.
- Do not heat or burn any of the materials (heat may release unknown fumes from paints or plastics).
- Handle sharp edges or rusty surfaces with care.

However, it is not only the scrap materials that are a concern. Substitutions or alterations of more standard materials also sometimes occur; what are the implications of making those changes? When starch is mixed with tempera paint to make finger paint, does it affect the non-toxicity of the paint? How does liquid soap or glycerin in tempera paint (to adhere it to slick or waxy surfaces) change the paint? Some teachers may add a preservative to tempera to keep it from going sour or to paste to keep it from becoming moldy. Of these preservatives, phenol, for example, is highly toxic, while oil of cloves is only slightly so. Even if the preservative used is not a serious hazard, what happens when it combines with other substances? Is the character of that substance changed? Might there be a synergistic effect (two combined materials creating an effect neither has alone)? Since the effects are not known, it is not advisable to make these alterations, even for economy. It would, at least, be wise to ask the manufacturer if they can provide information about what happens when these changes are made.

The inventiveness of art teachers knows few limits, and sometimes that is a hazard. Keep in mind that any certification of the non-toxicity of materials cannot be expected to hold true if they are altered by mixing them with other substances. Of what value is a toxic hazards identification program that may be undermined in this way?

Working with scrap materials and turning discards into art is exciting and provides worthwhile experiences for the children, but teachers must be sure unnecessary hazards are not brought into the classroom with the scraps. As with all such problems the teacher has two choices: not use the material at all, or treat it with the care and respect given known toxic substances.

Part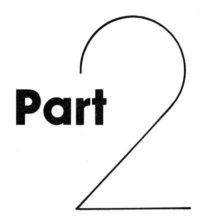

A CLOSER LOOK

5

Health Hazards in Detail

DEFINING TOXICITY

The word toxic is particularly difficult to pin down. Loosely defined, toxic means poison, but that is overly simplistic. A more accurate definition of toxicity is "a relative property of a chemical agent and refers to a harmful effect on some biologic mechanism and the condition under which this effect occurs" (McElroy, 1969, p. 1325). The key parts of this definition are the word "relative" and the phrase "condition under which this effect occurs." This means, essentially, that toxicity is not absolute and what might be fatal for one person in one set of circumstances might not be for another. Stated in yet another way, "In practical situations the critical factor is not the intrinsic toxicity of a substance per se but the risk or hazard associated with its use. Risk is the probability that a substance will produce harm under specified conditions." (Doull, 1980, p. 12).

Children under twelve are a "high risk" group because of their physical development. Also exposures causing serious reactions in some persons do not affect others as much or at all. These are examples of the relativity of toxicity and explain why just knowing the toxicity of a particular substance is not sufficient to safeguard students.

Toxicity rating information is extremely important, but knowing students, knowing the duration of exposure and knowing the extent of

42

the exposures are also important to a complete understanding of the possible harmful effects of materials. Above all, know whether conditions in the artroom are such that the teacher or students will be harmed by exposure to any of the substances used.

KNOW YOUR MATERIALS

Too often it does not occur to teachers that art materials may cause health problems. When a student — not always in an elementary grade — spreads the paste on the paper with his finger and then licks off the residue, the teacher's reaction is usually to say "don't do that!" But that reaction is probably more because the act is socially offensive than from concern that it might make anyone sick. Sometimes, however, putting some kinds of materials into the mouth, breathing them or even touching them can have serious results. For example, teachers should know that:

- Wallpaper paste often contains toxic preservatives.
- Vapors from permanent felt markers are toxic and repeated exposure can result in serious gastric and nervous system damage as well as liver damage.
- Batik wax vapors are flammable and can ignite at temperatures within the range of an ordinary hotplate; overheating also releases irritating fumes.
- Nearly all the chemicals used in photographic processing can cause skin, eye, lung or respiratory tract irritation or allergic reactions.

In selecting materials for the classroom, the teacher has several obligations concerning the potential health problems. First, learn as much as possible about the materials used in art processes and know whether they have any inherent harmful qualitities. Second, using a form such as that in Figure 8, find out whether students have any special health problems that might be aggravated by exposure to these materials or allergic reactions to the substances they might be using. And third, carefully and correctly instruct students in the use and handling of the materials. Obviously, the teacher's overall supervision in the classroom must insure that all materials are used as they should be.

Dear Parents:

During this year, we will be working with a variety of materials and processes in our art classes. We make every effort to insure that the materials are not harmful to students, but occasionally someone has an allergy or special sensitivity to something we do not know about. Will you please provide the information requested below so that we can avoid any unnecessary problems?

Date: _____

My (son) (daughter) has known allergies: Yes _____ No _____

My (son) (daughter) is allergic to the following substances:

_____

_____

If my son or daughter is exposed to a material to which he or she shows a previously unsuspected allergic reaction, please follow these instructions:

_____

_____

My phone number: _____

My doctor's phone number: _____

Signed: _____

Figure 8.

LABEL INFORMATION

There is little reason to be concerned with the health impact of materials that are not specifically used in the artroom. Broad knowledge about the hazards of art materials certainly can be useful in making decisions about new activities, but it is not critical. It may be distracting in the first stages of identifying art hazards. Go through the supply cabinets and be sure samples of everything there are set out for examination. Crayons, tempera paint, watercolors, felt markers, pencils, adhesives, solvents, inks and all other products need to be looked at. Include an example of each material from each manufacturer, and spend enough time reading (and making notes from) the label information to get a good understanding of what is there. Art supply cupboards often yield some very old, long out-of-use products. They should be discarded both because they may have deteriorated and because label information may be inaccurate. Sometimes old materials can be dangerous. For example, a product called Fibro-clay, produced by Milton-Bradley in the 1950s, contained asbestos. When research disclosed the cancer risks to asbestos, the product was immediately recalled. But it is still found in some artroom supplies and may yet be used by a teacher who discovers it in the back of the storage area and is unaware of its problems. Usually one of three different types of label information is available, and each presents some problem in interpretation.

Non-toxic Statements

Materials identified as non-toxic ought to be the safest to use, and generally they are. However, materials may be labeled non-toxic under provisions of the Federal Hazardous Substances Act if they are not acutely (immediately) toxic. This label statement alone does not address any long term effects the materials may have.

On the other hand, in the case of the non-toxic certification and testing program of the Art and Craft Materials Institute, "no product can earn the **CP** [Certified Product] or **AP** [Approved Product] seal if it contains any ingredient or known sensitizer that would produce an acute *or chronic* effect" (Deborah Fanning, Art and Craft Materials Institute, personal communication). These seals are authorized only for products which have been submitted to the institute for evaluation by an independent toxicologist.

The formulae are studied to determine if anything in the contents would be harmful to children even if ingested. If not, the product may display the seal.

From time to time, individual samples of these products are randomly taken from dealers and subjected to reexamination to insure there has been no formula change since the initial testing. This would justify withdrawal of the approval. The difference between CP and AP has to do with the quality of the materials and not with toxicity. Manufacturers also voluntarily provide warning labels on the number of products listing any chronic or long-term effects.

How should label information be interpreted? In general, let good sense be the guide. Feel reasonably comfortable using non-toxic materials, but don't be careless. Don't work with them in a poorly ventilated room (which is never a very pleasant experience anyway). Don't let students put even non-toxic materials in their mouths; it is a bad habit that may carry over into the use of other more harmful materials. Have students frequently wash their hands. Keep solvent or adhesive containers closed when they aren't actually being used. Clean up dust regularly with a wet mop or vacuum. Some students may be allergic even to non-toxic materials so watch for any special reactions, and, if there are any, get advice from the school nurse or call the parents for information.

Wordy, Technical Labels

Label information on occasion is very complete and provides a list of the specific chemical content. Even the concentrations of chemicals in the product are sometimes given. This information combined with other product warnings allows the teacher to anticipate problems and devise the best ways to avoid them. Should a student be accidentally exposed, product content information can facilitate handling the emergency.

If there is any question about the safety of the contents of a specific product, contact either the nearest poison control center or the Center for Occupational Hazards in New York and ask about it. If they are unable to reassure you, don't use the material.

Art teachers are usually not experienced in chemistry and should, therefore, not make assumptions about the contents of art materials. Seek help from people who deal with chemicals. If that is not possible, avoid questionable materials. In any case, avoid using art materials that require highly technical content data. If there is an important reason for using such materials, obtain expert advice on setting up procedures to protect students.

Labels Without Information

This type label creates the most difficult problem in evaluation, because some teachers assume that if no warning is stated, there is nothing to worry about in using the material. Wrong! Manufacturers are not required to disclose contents. Materials without label information are, therefore, potentially more hazardous than those with the most dire warnings. There is no sure way to tell about the possible dangers of unlabeled materials. When no content information or warning is provided, it is best routinely to treat the materials as hazardous. In general:

- Don't use unlabeled materials with elementary age children.
- Use unlabeled materials with older students only if there is good general room ventilation.
- Keep all materials covered when not actually in use.
- Store the materials carefully and in small quantities in places where they won't get knocked to the floor, broken, spilled or inadvertently opened and used.
- See that the material isn't put into mouths and that students frequently wash their hands.

The teacher should also request a "Material Safety Data Sheet" (OSHA Form 20) from the manufacturer and, if necessary, have it interpreted by an environmental or public health officer or a poison control center technician. This will reveal any special precautions that must be taken. If such persons are not available, do not use the material. If the safety data sheet is not provided, dispose of the material and don't use it again. If for some reason it absolutely must be used, always treat it as though it is extremely hazardous. Often suspicions about these materials will be unfounded and the precautions unnecessary, but for the students' sake, err on the safe side in decisions of this sort.

HOW MATERIALS AFFECT THE BODY

Acute injury provokes obvious body reactions. Cuts usually bleed; a smashed finger causes immediate pain and swelling and, before long, a blackened fingernail; touching a hot stove reddens or blisters the skin. In an even more dramatic example, a person swallowing poison will be immediately sick and may even die. Action is taken immediately because symptoms are seen or felt.

But all hazards are not this obvious. What happens internally may be hidden and often does not produce any noticeable symptoms until it is too late to take corrective action. There are many familiar examples of this: lung cancer and emphysema which often develop after long periods of smoking; cirrhosis of the liver which can be brought on by alcoholism; and, even more common, periodontal disease which develops because of inadequate mouth care and bacteria removal. By the time the symptoms of these serious illnesses are recognized, the condition is sometimes beyond help. These are known as chronic reactions.

Art teachers should understand how chemicals from art materials can enter the body, what happens when they do and what can be done to eliminate or reduce acute or chronic effects. With repeated exposure over time, some substances accumulate in the body. Teachers, who subject themselves to these materials on a regular basis, should be particularly concerned. While students may work with these materials for a few hours a week for several months, teachers usually work with them many hours daily for many years.

Even though there are no immediately visible effects, it can be assumed that if a hazardous substance is found in the artroom, anyone coming into contact with it will suffer some damage. The only sure prevention is to entirely eliminate contact with the substance. Knowing how these chemicals enter the body and the extent to which they are harmful will help in making decisions about whether to continue their use in the art program.

There are three ways foreign substances enter the body, and each provides access to vital organs and systems. Although the human body has a marvelous and complex defense mechanism, it can be breached and overloaded. It is the overload that must be prevented.

Skin Absorption (Contact)

The skin is an important part of the body's defense, but it can break down with exposure to certain substances, such as acids, caustic materials, solvents and bleaches. This is especially true when cuts or abrasions are present. Rashes, blistering, itching or flaking of the skin can result. Other damaging substances can enter the bloodstream and quickly move on to other parts of the body.

Some art materials may be sensitizers which, in certain persons, initiate allergies which did not previously exist. These can become increasingly severe with each subsequent exposure. Although desensitization shots sometimes help, there appears to be no sure way to reverse this effect. To insure these problems do not occur, it would be necessary to avoid any contact with such substances. If, however, the materials must be used in some essential processes, hands should be protected either with gloves that are resistant to the particular chemicals or with barrier creams which help shield the skin for up to four hours. These creams must always be re-applied after hands have been washed and care should be taken that the correct type of cream is used for the materials being handled.

Inhalation

Large particles of inhaled dust will be trapped to a great extent in the mucus of the nose or in the upper respiratory system. However, fumes, vapors, gases and most fine dust particles are not usually stopped by this "first line of defense," and some of them (those from overheated plastics, from glacial acetic acid used as a stop bath in photography, and from welding, for example) can irritate and damage the lining of breathing passages and lungs. Once in the lungs, these chemicals may burn the air sac tissue and eventually can cause chronic lung problems (McCann, 1979, p. 310). Prolonged exposure may cause bronchitis and emphysema which are aggravated by the effects of tobacco smoke, auto emission fumes and other pollutants in the air.

Some dusts, such as free silica in clay powder, can lead to silicosis or pulmonary fibrosis. Powder forms of fiber reactive (cold water) dyes or vapors from turpentine and epoxy hardeners may cause respiratory allergies or asthma.

Generally, it is possible to avoid using most of these materials without damaging the art program, but some, such as clay, must be included. Short of total elimination, anything which creates air borne fumes and particles must be controlled. It is imperative to plan for a separation of the mixing and working activities, to use correctly selected dust masks, and to provide good ventilation. (Adequate ventilation requires special considerations which are discussed in Chapter Three.) At the very least, however, cans of solvents, inks and adhesives must be kept closed when not actually in use, and floors need to be frequently wet-mopped—sweeping or dry mopping raises dust and does more harm than good.

Ingestion

Ingestion extends beyond the obvious example of young children eating paste. It more often occurs indirectly any time the mouth is touched by hands or tools carrying contaminants. A pensive moment, when fingers unconsciously touch the lips, is enough to transfer traces of some materials. "Pointing" a brush with the mouth is another example of indirect ingestion.

Except for swallowing vast amounts of material (an unlikely accident in a classroom), most substances enter the body through absorption from the stomach. The bloodstream transports contaminants to the liver for detoxification or to the kidneys for filtering. But harmful substances can overwork and damage those organs (as alcohol causes cirrhosis of the liver). The body then cannot cleanse itself of its own toxic products, to say nothing of foreign substances. Remember, the effects of many substances are cumulative and therefore can be quite serious. Even small ingested amounts must be avoided. Simple but regular practices such as washing hands, keeping them away from the mouth and not biting fingernails (to avoid picking up what may be lodged under them) will reduce possible ingestion. However, the only really effective control is to be constantly aware of how students work and be alert for any incidents of mouth contact with art materials.

HEALTH INSTRUCTION AND SUPERVISION

The best way for students to learn to use materials correctly is to give clear and careful instructions when they first encounter materials in the art class. This is especially true if students have previously adopted careless work habits. Allow ample time for this instruction when planning lessons. It is inefficient and ineffective to hurry through health hazards instruction in order to get into the project work more quickly—students will be unlikely to retain much, and the necessity for frequent reminders later on will interrupt the flow of class time.

Knowing about materials, being aware of student health problems and enforcing proper work habits are key to safe classroom procedures. There is no substitute for these in the effort to protect students from harmful interactions with art materials and processes.

6

Specific Safety Hazards

THE SAFETY ENVIRONMENT

The general conditions existing in the artroom set the stage for careful or careless work habits. To overlook these conditions is to overlook the basis of many hazards. Adequate space, appropriate storage and good housekeeping produce the safest working conditions. Sloppy work areas do more to cause accidents than almost anything else, but the effective management of all materials, equipment and work in progress will overcome this problem. Each of the following areas should be evaluated regularly.

Floors

Floors are often overlooked in classroom safety. Normally a classroom is on one level. But if the room is shared with other disciplines or is an old room that has been assigned artroom duty, there may be changes in level such as steps, platforms or risers. If so, the edges of these should be clearly marked with contrasting color for good visibility. Because changes in level are not usually under teacher control, traffic paths should be established well away from them if possible. Irregular changes are more likely to cause tripping or falling than just the change itself. In any case, it is important to reduce the use of any area where such changes occur.

Floors should be kept dry and non-slippery and anything spilled on them should be cleaned up at once. For instance, spilled water around the sink should not be allowed to puddle and should periodically be wiped dry during the class period. Students at any grade level should accept this responsibility but also know when to call for the teacher's help.

Custodians should be notified when floors develop cracks, loose or broken tiles or torn or frayed carpeting, any of which can trip people. If woodworking or wood sculpture projects are done in the room, be aware that wood chips and sawdust can increase the chance of slipping, especially on wooden floors. Keep floors clean by using a damp mop or shop type vacuum cleaner. Avoid sweeping, especially when students are in the room, since it raises dust and usually succeeds only in rearranging much of the waste materials; sweeping compounds are generally expensive and ineffective in controlling dust. If the floor is particularly slippery, especially around equipment or in worn places, report the condition to the school principal. Request that it be treated with a paint preparation containing abrasive particles or covered with non-slip adhesive strips where students stand or walk.

Plumbing

For some processes, particularly any which require acids or solvents, emergency washing facilities should be close to the working area. If a student is splashed with these substances, it is necessary to immediately flush the exposed parts of the body with water. To do this effectively, the proper equipment must be available; in some cases, this will mean an overhead shower. Often, however, a sink equipped with a flexible hose and spray attachment is an acceptable substitute for a drench hose since the chance of a serious splash in most artrooms is slight. Eyewash fountains or water faucets with inexpensive eyewash fittings should be located in any areas where acids are used. If there is no water source in the immediate area, portable eyewash stations containing at least five gallons of water will serve the purpose. They must be checked regularly for contamination. Such equipment should be at the proper height for the students who might need it.

An often overlooked plumbing hazard is the hot water temperature at the sink. If the temperature is erratic, students can unexpectedly receive scalding hot water. This situation should be reported to the custodian, but warnings and reminder signs at the sink may be necessary if the problem cannot be corrected.

Lighting

Certainly, all areas of the room must be well lighted, but no specific amount of light can insure safety. Generally, work surfaces with a dull, light finish will improve visibility and reduce glare. Some equipment, such as a jig saw, requires local, direct lighting; it should be placed so as not to be distracting or shine in the operator's eyes.

Adequate light not only improves visibility in working areas but helps to prevent tripping over unseen objects. Poor lighting cannot be justified on the basis of energy conservation; such false economy is not worth the risk of injury.

Room Size

Activities should properly correspond to classroom size. It is poor policy to expect students to work at any art activity unless the space is completely adequate. Overcrowding should not be permitted. School administrators sometimes consider it "efficient" space utilization to confine a relatively small art class to a small room, but the trade-off may well be the unnecessary injury of a student. Curriculum planning which calls for activities that crowd the space available is also poor policy. If the room size cannot be adjusted, the curriculum has to be.

Furniture should be arranged so students can work without being impeded. Many tools and some materials require space for arm swinging (as with hammers) and broad, sweeping movement (as with wire manipulation). The arrangement of participants needs to be organized accordingly. Be sure too that space between work tables is kept clear of obstructions and allows for easy movement through the room. The movement of students and materials or equipment around the room should be limited and carefully planned. Be sure also that the room arrangement allows for an easy exit in the event of an emergency.

Storage

Adequate storage in the artroom should be provided for bulk supplies, materials in use and partially completed projects. Providing this storage space prevents cluttering and allows for easy movement. Contending with a crowded working area will promote careless work habits among students. Constant reshuffling of materials to clear work space is annoying and can cause impatience which may lead to accidents.

Art teachers are notorious collectors of materials of all kinds that may prove useful for future projects. No one advocates arbitrary or wasteful disposal of such materials, but these "collectibles" must be neatly stacked or boxed and stored in areas completely out of normal traffic patterns or work areas. A periodic culling of such materials should take place—any materials that have not been used in a year probably never will be.

Noise

Power tools which are used frequently will create a disturbing level of noise in the room. It may be necessary to restrict the times they may be used and to require students working with them to wear hearing protection. Ear plugs or industrial type ear muffs will significantly reduce the potential for hearing loss.

ARTROOM ORDER

The myth that mess, sometimes called "creative chaos," makes for better art has permeated many artrooms. It results in the frequent loss of tools and equipment tossed out by accident, or waste of materials, such as torn or dirty paper or contaminated and dried up paint. It also makes for very unsafe working conditions.

Actually, there is little reason to believe creativity is enhanced in any way by a messy work area. The irritation of having to search for tools lost amidst clutter is hardly conducive to exciting and innovative art work. Nor does the waste and carelessness seem likely to have any positive effect on the quality of art. In fact, the free and ready access to tools and materials characteristic of an orderly environment probably enhances the free atmosphere of the work area and allows for greater creativity.

Sometimes these "ordinary" safety hazards are overshadowed by the more "exotic" problems such as getting rid of chemical fumes. But it isn't very sensible to worry about adequate ventilation and at the same time forget that serious injuries can occur from tripping over materials that are obstructing traffic. The fact that the carelessly stacked cans of paint which have crashed down on someone's head contain non-toxic paint is of no consequence in this case.

There are several obvious reasons for maintaining the artroom in good order. Some points have to do with safety, others with economics, but all relate to developing and sustaining an atmosphere which encourages art production. Be aware that:

- Properly stored tools remain in good condition longer, and tools in good condition are less likely to cause accidents.
- Dirty floors tend to be slicker than clean floors. Bits of paper, and particularly sawdust, reduce traction and increase the chances of slipping, especially on waxed floors.
- Carelessly stacked materials invite problems; it sometimes becomes necessary to pull paper from the bottom of the stack and the results of that are obvious to anyone who has tried it.
- Trying to work on litter-strewn tables or desks reduces effective control over tools and equipment, leading to careless actions. School books should always be put well out of the way of working or walking areas.

Keeping an orderly artroom isn't very exciting, but it is absolutely necessary in any classroom safety program. Doing so demonstrates to students that proper care of equipment and material is the key to a good working environment. If no litter and dust are allowed to accumulate, it is easier to find effective methods of controlling other hazards. For example, keeping the clay storage and mixing room in meticulous order reduces dust control problems—wet-mopping can, then, take care of most of the dust, and less of it has to be exhausted by mechanical devices.

The teacher must have a positive attitude toward an orderly working environment and storage areas; fortunately, it is one which doesn't have to wait for special budget action. Perhaps even more important, it shows a concern that will help convince administrators when there is need for special equipment to combat other types of hazards. When a teacher shows that everything possible is being done to eliminate hazards, administrators are more likely to provide funds to do the rest.

WORKING WITH TOOLS

Clear instructions must be given when the equipment is first used, and those instructions must be followed. Correcting the student when the equipment is being used improperly and helping the student develop the right habits are also part of the teacher's role. The simplest tool has the potential to cause serious injury, and it is often familiar tools that cause problems. What are the functions of the most typical tools and what determines necessary instruction?

Cutting

Most tools in the artroom fall into this category. Scissors, paper cutter, saws, knives, wood and linoleum cutters, metal snips and wire cutters are all common, and all require special initial instruction along with frequent reminders about correct use.

- Do not assume the students know how to handle and correctly use any cutting tools, even those with which they ought to be the most familiar.
- Give careful instruction and supervision for blunt scissors just as for pointed ones to insure good habits for all types of scissors. Do not assume that blunt scissors are any less dangerous than pointed ones.
- Use the proper tool for the job. Do not, for example, cut wire with metal snips or scissors, cord or string with wire cutters, wood with linoleum cutters or cardboard with the paper cutter. To do so dulls the tool and makes it unreliable when used for its proper purpose.
- Keep cutting tools sharp. Dull or chipped blades slip easily and cause painful cuts. If necessary, have sharpening done professionally, or discard the tool—it is false economy to continue using a tool in poor condition. It is good economy to teach students how to sharpen tools themselves.
- Store tools so as to protect them and in a way that makes distribution easy and safe: scissors in scissor holders, drawers for knives, racks for saws and metal and wire cutters.
- Set up controlled distribution procedures that minimize handling of tools.

- Establish specific work spaces for any power tools.
- Severely limit and personally supervise student use of the paper cutter and be sure the blade spring is always functioning. If possible, substitute a rotary trimmer for a guillotine-type cutter; injuries are far less likely to occur.
- Be sure that any material being cut is held securely: vises and clamps should be available when needed and students should know how to use them.

Piercing

Although not done as often as cutting, piercing materials is even more hazardous because it involves sharply pointed tools such as punches, awls, drills, scissors and compasses. Puncture wounds to hands, fingers, legs or eyes are not uncommon in piercing activities. Careful supervision and small groups are necessary. Hand drills are probably the least dangerous piercing tools to use, provided they are sharp so as to reduce slipping and used with the correct bit. A vise to hold the material is absolutely necessary if the drilling is done into a rounded or irregular surface.

Pounding

Hammers and mallets should always be used appropriately. Obviously, wood or rubber mallets shouldn't be used to pound nails, and steel hammers shouldn't be used to hammer-print linoleum blocks. But this has more to do with damage to the tools or to the work than with safety. However, damaged tools will not function well when they are used later. Be aware, too, that hammers come in different weights. They should not be too heavy for the student or the job for which they are used.

Squeezing and Pinching

The tools used in these processes are not especially dangerous, providing reasonable care is exercised to be sure fingers are not caught in them. Pliers, vises and printing presses are usually the only tools used for these purposes and simple instructions should be sufficient. However, a printing press usually has rollers and a moving bed, and instructions should be particularly clear about these danger areas on the press.

Heating

Processes such as batik, wax encaustic, printing on fabric, welding or soldering require hotplates, irons or butane or other type torches. These are potentially very dangerous both because of direct burns and because they are often used to apply heat to very flammable materials. Use low temperature and double boilers for melting waxes, and closely supervise and control the use of torches. Be aware of the flash point temperature of wax used for batik; use candy thermometers to maintain a safe margin. Burns are among the most painful and disfiguring injuries. Every effort must be made to prevent them and to know how to treat them if they do occur. Welding tanks must be chained to prevent them from falling over and rupturing or damaging the gauges; welding hoses must be kept clear of any regularly used areas where they might cause tripping.

Power Tools

Power tools are increasingly common in artrooms: the prices of electric drills, drill presses, band saws, sabre saws and sanders are more and more within the reach of art budgets. The same precautions concerning the use of hand saws and drills are appropriate for power equipment of any type:

- Keep all tools in good condition.
- Use sharp blades and bits and store the tools properly with the bits and blades removed.
- Carefully instruct and supervise the use of the tools.
- Set aside specific places for power tools to be used.
- Use three-pronged, grounded extension cords. Completely disconnect free standing tools from the power source when not in use.

There may be other tools and equipment which have not been specifically mentioned here, and each teacher must see that students know, understand, respect and properly use any of them.

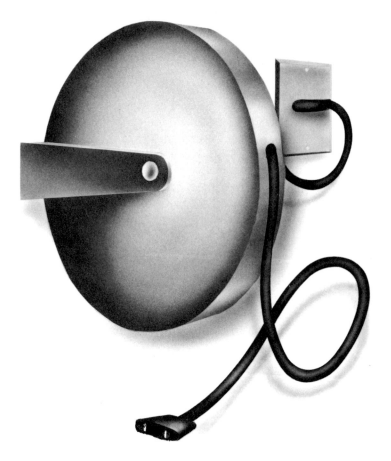

Extension cords and hoses should be placed so they are not tripped over, causing hot spills or pulling things from tables. Electric cords on retracting reels, hanging above the work area for easy access, are a good solution to the problem of cords on the floor.

CLASSROOM SAFETY CHECK

Check-lists are the most effective way to control hazards. While most teachers may rightly feel that their teaching time is already seriously eroded by bookkeeping tasks of dubious importance, the time taken to make a conditions check can be very worthwhile. It is also a good way of involving students in a learning experience.

Safety checks should be regularly scheduled each week and rotated through the different classes to give all students the experience. If the students participate as "reporting monitors," it soon will be apparent to them that room and tool conditions are important. They will learn what to look for in identifying hazards. When they have learned to do this as a regularly scheduled activity, it will become second nature for them to notice and report any conditions which may seem hazardous. Awareness of safety conditions is best learned by the regular experience of monitoring those conditions. When a teacher demonstrates that safety is important enough to give it time and attention, the students will recognize it too. This is a valuable life-long attitude that will develop through this simple, helpful and regular classroom activity.

Use a form similar to the Safe Conditions Check (Figure 9) for recording the hazard information. It should include sufficient space to insure all important conditions can be noted and provide a way to indicate clearly when something needs to be corrected.

When a hazard is found, the teacher should correct it if possible or call it to the attention of the principal or custodian. By recording and reporting hazards information on a specific form, action is much more likely to occur than if the notification is made by an informal note or a casual comment in the hallway.

Not all aspects of safety can be easily checked by students. Certainly conditions of the room as well as tools and equipment within the room can be done by students. But what about safety as it relates to procedures, work habits or the thoroughness of safety instruction the teacher gives? Since there are no "safety examiners" who can evaluate teacher performance, it will be very difficult to get observations which are reliable. The task thus falls to the teachers themselves. Several points should be reviewed on a regular basis:

- Are safety notations included in all lesson plans?

- Are regular and consistent instructions given for working procedures and tool use, even for tools frequently used?
- Are the students' work habits monitored? Are corrective comments made and is appropriate behavior demanded?

To determine how well the students are learning, evaluate and record the overall manner in which they work by using a form similar to the Performance and Attitudes Toward Safety (Figure 10). When they are working on an activity in which specific safety procedures are to be followed, use this form to record how they work. It is a good idea to check them from a location in the room away from usual observation points; stand at the back or side of the room so as to have a fresh perspective and reduce the chance of overlooking details. In addition, it may be helpful to ask the principal, a fellow teacher or a teacher aide to use the Performance and Attitudes Toward Safety form and to share with you their observations of the class. This not only provides an outsider's view but also helps these people become aware of safety practices in your classroom. Having such a visitor should not be seen as a threat and is a way of being sure that important safety practices are reflected in the way the students work when observed by others.

SAFETY CONDITIONS CHECK		
Room number: _____		
Teacher: _____ Date: _____		

General	O.K.	Needs attention (comment)
Floor condition		
Lights		
Aisles clear		
Storage area		
Ventilation		
Windows open easily		
Exhaust fans working		
Tools		
Hand tools in good order		
Power tools in good order		
Electric cords		
Tool storage		
Materials		
Well organized storage		
Solvents properly stored		

Added Comments

Submitted to principal: _____ date: _____
(teacher signature)

Principal Acknowledgment: _____ date: _____
(principal signature)

Figure 9.

PERFORMANCE AND ATTITUDES TOWARD SAFETY

Room: _____

Teacher: _____ Date: _____

Performance	O.K.	Needs Attention (comment)
Work area orderly		
Tools used correctly		
Materials well organized		
Distribution efficient		
Collection well done		
Tools properly stored		
Eye protection worn as needed		
Hair kept out of way		
Instructions understood		
Attitude		
Tools well cared for		
Attention to work (no horseplay)		
Concern about work habits		
Reminders necessary		

Comments

Teacher or observer's name _____ date: _____
Teacher initials _____ date: _____

Figure 10.

7

Hazards of Common Art Activities

Not all art activities are hazardous enough to warrant special attention. However, many important art activities do involve materials and processes that present unusual problems in health and safety. Some use chemicals or tools that are especially hazardous. They are "special hazards" and need to be well understood.

All of these activities are important to a comprehensive art program and should not be discontinued because of their potential danger. Rather, the problems should be recognized and minimized. Students should be properly instructed so they can benefit from the experiences yet not be subject to risk. With concern and careful planning this is certainly possible.

DRAWING

To most teachers, drawing seems to be one area where there are few problems of health or safety. Usually this is true. For most students, working with crayons, markers, pencils, pen and ink, charcoal, brush washes or pastels are activities that cause few problems. (Obviously, attention must always be given to the handling of sharp tools such as pencils and pens to be sure they are used safely.)

Some exceptions exist:

- The most serious problem is from aerosol spray fixatives used for charcoal and pastel, which should be used only with extremely good ventilation or preferably outdoors. It is no solution to use spray fixative in the hall outside the artroom, since that will contaminate the entire school. Also, charcoal and pastels usually create large quantities of dust in the artroom which can irritate some students.
- Only water-based markers are to be used. The dangers inherent in permanent markers have been discussed earlier.
- Check oil crayons carefully. Many are imported and the non-toxic label may not be entirely accurate. Use only oil crayons that carry the AP (Approved Product) or CP (Certified Product) seal of the Art and Craft Materials Institute.

PAINTING

Regardless of the type of painting done in the artroom, some pigments should always be suspect. While most pigments are non-toxic, there are a number of toxic inorganic pigments which should be avoided. Seeger (1982) and McCann (1985) cite the following:

Naples Yellow (Antimony)
Cobalt Violet (Arsenic)
All cadmium pigments (Cadmium)
Chromium Oxide Green, Veridian, Chrome Yellow, Zinc Yellow, Strontium Yellow (Chromium)
Cobalt Blue, Cobalt Green, Cobalt Yellow, Cerulean Blue, Cobalt Violet (Cobalt)
Flake White, Naples Yellow, Chrome Yellow (Lead)
Manganese Blue, Raw Umber, Burnt Umber, Mars Brown, Manganese Violet (Manganese)
Vermillion, Cadmium Vermillion Red (Mercury)

Many of these are corrosive to the skin and cause irritation of respiratory tract, mucous membranes. They also produce allergic reactions. Precautions in the use of these pigments will reduce problems and so will good housekeeping, keeping food out of the studio and careful personal hygiene (frequent hand washing, for example). Brushes should never be put in the mouth.

Unless a class is working with these specific pigments, the greatest hazards in painting will come from turpentine or other toxic solvents. Obviously if the painting medium is acrylic, watercolor or tempera where the solvent is water, that hazard doesn't exist. In actuality, the use of oil paint is virtually indefensible in any public school art program. Because oil painting requires toxic solvents and possibly toxic pigments and is nearly always done in areas with poor ventilation, it should be avoided in the high school and never done in elementary or junior high school.

Sometimes students or parents feel that oil painting represents the highest and most advanced form of art and want it in the school for reasons of prestige. Teachers should not be misled by that viewpoint; there is little that can be done in oil paint that can't be done equally well in acrylics. Eliminating the need for turpentine and paint thinners more than compensates for the small loss in visual quality that might result. There is nothing significantly special to be learned about painting through the use of oils to justify either the trouble or expense to make them safe to work within the classroom.

PRINTMAKING

Both health and safety hazards can be significant in printmaking. Careful instructions and procedures will minimize them. Health problems include exposure to inks, solvents and acids, while the safety concerns relate primarily to injuries resulting from the use of cutting tools and the crushing action of various parts of the printing presses.

The health problems are most easily solved at the elementary printmaking levels because hazardous materials and processes can be eliminated; the safety hazards are most easily solved at the advanced levels by simple but thorough instructions. Safety must be the major target at the elementary level, since children are still learning skills required with tools. At the secondary level, health hazards resulting from exposures to the chemicals in inks and solvents are difficult to deal with and may present serious problems for students who come into contact with them.

Beginning Printmaking

Found objects, vegetables, glue, cardboard and linoleum are the materials most used to make prints; tempera, finger paint and water-based blockprinting ink are most often used to print them in the most introductory print courses. Safety hazards here primarily involve the tools used to cut the surface of the image carrier or block. As always, there is no substitute for good planning, careful instruction and continuous monitoring of the way students are working. To minimize problems:

- Limit beginning students to working with relief or simple stencil prints. There is a sufficient variety of these experiences to provide many printmaking opportunities without attempting other processes. Water-based silk screen can be used with junior high or middle school students, but these students should be sufficiently advanced in the silk screen process to justify the cost of these expensive materials.
- Be sure all tools fit the age, size and muscle control of students. Cutting a design into the slippery face of half a potato with a paring knife is no task for most children, and probably not for many adults either.
- Show students how to hold the cutting tool as well as their work so that when the tool slips (as it will), no harm is done.
- Sharp tools must be used so that cutting is sure, constant and predictable.
- Cutting activities must be kept separated from the printing area to reduce confusion and mess.
- Linoleum blocks must be cut only with linoleum cutting tools, and these tools used only for that purpose.
- Meticulous instructions must be given for any type of press, and children should work in pairs during the printing steps so that one can monitor as well as help the other.
- Improper practices must be immediately corrected.
- No horseplay can be allowed in the vicinity of cutting activities.

To keep health hazards to a minimum, be sure only water-based, non-toxic paint or ink is used. There is no need for solvents other than water with these inks; in fact, there is never any reason to use oil-based inks with children under twelve. The problems associated with oil-based materials and their solvents are far greater than any advantages of permanence or color quality. Blockprinting on fabric, which requires oil blockprinting inks or special textile inks or paint, should be delayed until junior or senior high.

Print processes offer a great variety of learning experiences and expressive possibilities, so printmaking should be encouraged and exploited. With thorough planning, good instructions and constant monitoring, the potential hazards of all of these processes can be effectively controlled. Because printmaking is a fairly complex activity, students can, at the same time, learn important lessons about responsibility so that hazards encountered later in the more advanced activities will be better understood and significantly reduced.

Advanced Printmaking

In junior and senior high school, many printmaking processes are the same as those in the elementary grades. Only the content and images become more complex, and skill levels increase. To this extent, the same hazards exist for older students and can be handled in the same manner. However permanence of the print may become more a part of the design concept (textile printing, or posters to be displayed outside, for example), or new processes such as silk screen or intaglio printing may be introduced. To make permanent block prints, oil-based inks and the solvents they require are necessary. While the hazards of these may be reduced by good housekeeping practices and careful instruction, they cannot be completely eliminated. The problems of course are that these oil-based inks and solvents produce harmful vapors which must be ventilated; can contaminate the skin which must be protected; are flammable so they must be properly stored; and produce waste materials that require special disposal.

To eliminate these problems, consider using water-soluble silk screen inks which are permanent and are also available in fluorescent and textile inks. These materials require only soap and water for clean-up. While silk screen produces visual effects very different from block printing, in general it is possible to develop designs which will be just as effective. The reduction of the hazards involved is worth the extra effort that will be required. Water-based substitution for intaglio processes is not possible and all precautions to protect the students from ink, solvent and acid exposure will have to be taken.

Solvent and Ink Fumes

The only effective way to control vapors is through proper ventilation. Most schools do not have adequate local exhaust systems for extensive printmaking programs and cannot afford them. As an alternative, keep solvent clean-up activities centralized to an area where air can be moved away from the students by a fan and open window system. Remember, however, this requires incoming air to make up what the fan blows out (and relying only on open windows also would always make printmaking a warm weather activity). Keep all solvent containers closed except when actually being poured, and do the pouring in a well ventilated area. Immediately put the solvent- and ink-soaked rags and paper into a closed waste container to contain the fumes. Strictly limit the number of students working in the print area at one time so that minimum amounts of ink and solvents are in use. If the odor of the solvent permeates the general classroom, the ventilation system is not working effectively—either the volume of air being moved must be increased or the number of students working at one time must be decreased.

Contamination by Skin Contact

This problem can be significantly reduced by using plastic gloves during all phases of the printing process. Gloves may seem clumsy at first, particularly for students with small hands. But with time, using them becomes quite natural and virtually eliminates the problem of ink or solvents coming into direct contact with the skin. The type of glove will determine its effectiveness. Almost any household plastic glove will protect from ink contamination. Gloves used with solvents must be more carefully selected and should not be expected to provide long term protection from heavy solvent contact. If the use is limited and the gloves are replaced frequently, significant protection can be expected. Careful disposal of dirty gloves, as with waste rags and paper, is a must.

Disposal

All waste paper and solvent soaked rags must go into self-closing covered waste cans, and these cans must be emptied daily. Whether the contents of these cans represent a sufficient quantity to require special waste disposal procedures is a matter for the school principal to determine in consultation with appropriate local health officials. The teacher should inform the principal that waste materials are being generated as part of regular art activities and request instructions about proper disposal. Waste solvents should not simply be washed down the sink drain, since that usually leads directly to city water treatment plants and can create serious pollution problems.

Unquestionably, there are problems to be solved in order to work with printmaking safely. However, these can be largely dealt with through careful teacher management, attention to procedures, thorough instruction and a plan of action for both teacher and students. The visual rewards of prints are such that teachers should have strong motivation to work out any problems and enforce their solutions. At the same time, this will help students learn the health and safety practices which need to be instituted. They are likely to carry these lessons with them throughout their lives. It isn't easy, but the results justify the effort.

FIBERS AND DYES

In general, the hazards involved in fiber work are not extreme, but two aspects of fiber work require some attention if health hazards are to be eliminated.

Bacteria, Dust, Fibers

The first of these is perhaps easier to handle; it involves working with the carding, spinning, and weaving of various fibers. In most schools, yarns are purchased commercially, and concern about bacterial contamination is virtually unnecessary, since these materials can be expected to be free of problems. However, when wool or other fibers are used in spinning, be sure the raw fiber has been thoroughly sanitized. Contamination by this means is rare but has occurred and can be very serious. It is a problem simply avoided. Do not work with any raw wool, for example, which has been brought into this country "informally."

Working with jute rope or burlap in weaving or macrame projects can produce very irritating airborne fiber or dust particles which may aggravate or even cause respiratory problems in some students. Wearing an inexpensive dust mask will reduce these problems significantly.

Dyeing

The second aspect of fiber work that creates potential health hazards is working with dyes. There are a great variety of dyes available which are used in different processes and for different fabrics. Unfortunately, not a great deal is known about the potential problems associated with them. Recent studies have shown that food dyes, previously believed harmless, are now thought to be carcinogenic. Benzidine congener (family) dyes, used in many common products, have also been found to be carcinogenic and have been discontinued in some applications (NIOSH, 1983). Many other dyes and the chemicals used with them as mordants (particularly chrome, ammonia and oxalic acid) can cause various toxic reactions, including respiratory and eye irritation, skin corrosion and allergies. Part of the difficulty is that dyes are often re-packaged by distributors, and warning information that appears on the original packages is sometimes not transferred to the new container.

Fiber-reactive (cold water) dyes seem to be the most hazardous, causing symptoms such as asthma, "hay fever," swollen eyes and, after long exposure, sudden severe allergy (McCann, 1979, p. 333).

In all work with dyes, it is recommended that an approved dust mask and gloves be worn to reduce exposure. When mixing dye powder, use an entire package at one time so that leftover packages will not spill and release dust. McCann also suggests that when possible, the entire dye powder package be submerged in water while it is being opened to prevent any inhalation. He also suggests making a glove box. Shellac the inside of a cardboard box to seal it, put a glass or plexiglass sheet on the top to see through, and cut handholes in the sides. Wear gloves and mix the dye inside the box. No mask will be needed, and there is no messy clean-up required.

Tie-dyeing and batik are relatively common dyeing processes carried on at nearly all school levels. Common household dyes are often used in these processes, and they should be handled with great care. Wearing gloves is very important. Thoroughly wash any parts of the body on which the dyes have accidentally been spilled. Restrict mixing of dye from powder to students who have been carefully trained, since the ability to control this process will be limited.

Batik involves the use of heated wax which is highly flammable and can cause painful burns. Use only a double boiler set-up, where the wax is placed in a container which, in turn, stands in water to which the heat is applied. Never heat wax directly on a hot-plate which might accidentally be turned to an unsafe high temperature. In any dyeing process requiring the heating of the dye bath, exercise extreme care to prevent scalding.

Textile Printing

Both blockprinting or silk screen printing on textiles are popular activities with junior or senior high students. These processes allow a variety of craft activities, perhaps the most common of which is printing on T-shirts. For permanence, either an oil-based blockprinting or silk screen ink is often used, although these inks have the disadvantage of making the fabric stiff. Special textile inks, which leave the material soft, are often preferred. In either case, the inks themselves, and the solvents required to work them, create the same toxicity problems as in other print processes. Whether it is turpentine or a commercially prepared thinning oil, caution must be used to reduce skin contact and inhalation of the fumes. This means gloves or barrier creams, and good ventilation of the work area. The use of acrylic paints or inks is recommended as a substitute that eliminates most problems. Manufacturers of acrylic products may have suggestions for using their products in textile printing. Don't assume ink or paint must be petroleum based to be permanent.

As with so many processes, good housekeeping practices and common sense are fundamental to eliminating hazards associated with fiber work. In many cases, the problems mentioned here will not arise. Working with commercial yarns is the norm in most classes, and dyeing is usually a very limited activity. Exercising reasonable care, wearing dust masks and gloves when they are appropriate and being meticulous in instructing students about working procedures are usually sufficient. If more advanced processes are desired, the hazards of both dust and dye should be thoroughly researched with the intent of devising procedures to protect everyone.

STAINED GLASS

There are several glass fabricating processes generally referred to as stained glass, but only one of these, leaded glass, seems likely to be done in an artroom setting. Working with epoxy resins or concrete to fill the channels between very thick, faceted glass, or laminating glass panels into layers are processes more likely undertaken by artists specializing in this medium and should be done in schools only with very advanced instruction.

Leaded glass, however, is well within the skill levels of students at the junior and senior high levels. Attention needs to be given to those aspects of the process which can cause injury or long-term health problems.

Glass Cutting

It looks incredibly easy when done by an expert, but cutting glass often doesn't turn out quite like it should. At best, clean cuts leave very sharp edges that need to be smoothed with emery paper. Obviously, the glass must be handled with great care to avoid cuts. When the planned cut is less smooth than intended, and the trimming must be done with grozing pliers, extreme care should be taken in handling the glass. Not only are the edges of the glass likely to be jagged, but the small pieces and slivers of glass must be watched very carefully and contained as much as possible. Work should be done over a cleared, smooth surface so the fragments can be easily brushed into a waste container. Goggles must be worn to protect the eyes from any shards of glass that fly in unexpected directions. As each piece is cut, set it well out of the way so that it must be handled as little as possible before the assembling of the project.

Handling Lead Came

The **major** precaution necessary in handling the lead came, which holds the glass pieces together, is to be sure that hands and finger nails are thoroughly washed afterward. There is little problem with skin contact, but particles of lead, from cutting or sanding the came, can be passed to the mouth and ingested. If enough is ingested the typical problems associated with lead poisoning may result. Keep hands clean, and wipe the work surface frequently with a damp cloth.

Soldering

The solder used in leaded glass work is a 60–40 or 50–50 mixture of lead and tin and should not have an "acid core." In the soldering process, it is the solder which melts, not the lead came, and the lead fumes given off from that solder should not be breathed. Good general ventilation in the work area plus a fan that will blow the fumes away from the participants should be sufficient. A better method is to rig a vacuum cleaner with its intake near the work and the exhaust hose arranged to carry the fumes outside. If possible, work in front of an open window with an exhaust fan to extract fumes (McCann, p. 84). Do not solder under a canopy hood, since the fumes will be drawn up and directly past a student leaning over his or her work.

In general, wear gloves that will protect hands from being cut by sharp glass edges, yet still allow free manipulation of the glass. Limit cutting to simple shapes until good cutting skills have been achieved. Exercise care in the process of applying the putty, so that sharp edges of the came, particularly at joints, do not cause cuts.

Because of the manipulative skills required to cut or handle glass and the harmful cumulative effects of lead fumes, leaded glass work should not be undertaken until junior or senior high.

CERAMICS

In recent years, ceramics has become an increasingly popular art form. There are probably few schools where some ceramics activities don't occur and many where the program is extremely sophisticated and extensive. It is not only one of the most pervasive art activities in our society, it is one of the most complex. It involves a number of often ignored hazards.

From the raw material to the finished object, clay goes through several different states and a series of manipulations, each of which has inherent health or safety hazards. It is in three of these stages the most serious hazards occur: mixing, glazing and firing.

Clay Mixing

Normally, the digging and refining processes occur before teachers and students come into contact with clay, so the first problem usually encountered is with clay dust that escapes from the bags in which it is packaged. During commercial preparation, clay is ground very finely so that leakage from these bags is not uncommon. The bags sometimes are ripped in delivery, but more often they are torn open after arrival and partially used. As a result, the environment in which clay is stored is almost always a dusty place. This clay dust is then scuffed into the air and tracked throughout the school, leaving a film of powder over nearly everything in direct contact with it.

Silica may compose up to 60 percent of the clay. Usually it is chemically bonded with other elements, but, if not, it is known as free silica and can be the cause of chronic silicosis (Seeger, 1982, pp. 14–15). Silicosis is ultimately a disabling disease of the lungs. No one should be unnecessarily exposed to free silica; its effect is long-term and usually does not result in problems for 10–15 years. It is, however, the ceramics teacher and serious student, working with clay for a period of years, who are in the greatest jeopardy. For their protection, as well as for short-term students, correct clay handling and mixing procedures must be maintained. The teacher's own risk should be sufficient motivation to insure an effective program of dust containment.

In addition to the health hazards, the safest possible procedures for mixing clay must be devised. Pug mills and clay mixers should be used only after detailed instructions have been given and tested and always with close teacher supervision. Incidentally, be sure that barrels used to collect clay for reuse are frequently checked for foreign materials or small tools which may have been inadvertently dropped in. These could later create serious problems in the mixing equipment.

The following suggestions should be observed to limit clay mixing hazards as much as possible:

- Determine if the quantity of clay to be used warrants mixing it from powder. In the middle and junior high schools, the quantity needed often does not in most cases justify exposing the students to clay dust hazards. While it is somewhat more expensive, ready mixed clay is preferable because it eliminates the need for dust handling or mixing equipment. An explanation and demonstration of how clay is made will be sufficient until students are working at a more advanced level.
- Store and mix clay in an area separated from the studio so as to reduce the area of dust contamination.
- Keep all powdered clay bags in storage covered tightly with polyethylene sheeting in order to contain the dust.
- Stack clay bags off the floor on pallets or shelves so that cleaning the floor is easier and more complete.
- Wet mop the floor of the mixing area frequently; never sweep or dry mop, since this stirs up dust particles and provides inadequate cleaning. Vacuuming is effective only if there is a HEPA (high energy particulate air) filter in the vacuum cleaner which will prevent recycling of the dust through the air.
- Wear a dust mask specifically designed to filter out silica and other particles whenever working in the clay mixing room or when sanding a dry, but unfired (greenware) object. Be sure the mask is the correct type (one having NIOSH approval #TC-21C-132, for example).
- Have a local exhaust system operating whenever the clay mixer is in use; this will draw off most though not all of the problem particles.

Glazing

The second stage of clay work involves the process of glazing. This is a complex area, since the great variety of materials used in mixing glazes makes it difficult to generalize about the hazards.

Glazes are often purchased ready-mixed, but in some programs the teacher will have the students learn glaze formulations, using bulk glaze chemicals to mix their own colors. In either form, simple rules should govern their handling:

- Allow no food in the area where glazes are being used; it is very easy to contaminate that food and thereby ingest chemicals.
- Always use a stirring stick; never use hands to mix the glaze.
- Wash hands thoroughly after working with the glaze.
- Work on an easily cleanable surface when applying the glaze; formica or plastic are suitable. Clean with a wet sponge or rag when finished.
- Glazes should be sprayed only in a booth with an exhaust fan that effectively carries away excess airborne particles.

When mixing the glazes from powder, there is the additional need to exercise extreme care containing the dust. This means there should be effective local ventilation or that toxic dust masks or respirators must be worn during the mixing process. Protective clothing such as a smock or shop coat should also be worn during this process. To contain dust, wear these garments only in the mixing area; wash them frequently. Figure 11 lists several glaze substances that should *not* be used in a school setting; all are suspected carcinogens or highly toxic.

Perhaps the most recognized of glaze hazards is lead. But it is sometimes used in classrooms. The usual justification for this is that the objects being glazed will not be used as food containers, and thus there will be no chance of contamination. Two factors need to be considered, however. First, if any other objects are fired along with lead-glazed pieces, they are likely to be contaminated by lead fumes (as is the air around the kiln during firing). Thus the lead can be passed along in sufficient quantities to represent a hazard to ultimate users of the objects.

Second, lead frits, often thought to be non-soluble and therefore safe for use, may not always be so. "Lead frits vary in solubility (the capacity to dissolve in liquids to form a solution) depending on factors like: method of production, size of particles. Due to the variation in solubility some inhaled and ingested particles may dissolve in body fluids. Therefore, we believe that lead frits are not reliably non-toxic and should be handled with the same precautions used for other lead compounds. . . . Copper used in, or on, ware fired in a kiln with lead containing objects can affect the solubility of the lead on other ware" (Seeger, p. 32). Although there may be some justification for professional potters to use these materials in their private studios, there can be no such justification for their use in a school setting.

GLAZE MATERIALS WHICH SHOULD *NOT* BE USED IN SCHOOL CERAMICS PROGRAMS[1,2]

The following materials are suspected carcinogens or are highly toxic and, regardless of how carefully they may be handled, should not be used in junior or senior high school settings. While it might be possible to control them in the studio of a professional potter or even the studio of a very limited number of advanced college students, there is no justification for subjecting secondary level students to the inherent hazards.

Lead and its compounds: (-acetate, -silicate, -bisilicate, -monoxide, -oxide)

Arsenic and its compounds: (-oxide, white oxide, -trioxide)

Cadmium and its compounds: (-oxide, -sulfide, -chloride)

Nickel and its compounds: (may produce highly toxic nickel carbonyl in firing)

Beryllium and its compounds (-oxide, beryl, beryllia)

Zinc chromate

Selenium and its compounds (-oxide, -dioxide)

Any uranium compounds

---

1. Barazani, *CAA Studio Guide,* pp. 19–20.
2. Seeger, pp. 27–35.

Figure 11.

Firing

The final step in the ceramics process which involves hazards to teachers and students is kiln firing. It involves intense heat around the kiln, and the vitrifying clay or glazes give off a variety of fumes, some of which may be highly toxic. All kiln firing, for example, produces carbon monoxide when various impurities in the clay decompose during firing. Depending on the clay and glaze content, gases such as sulfur dioxide, fluorine, chlorine and nitrogen oxides are produced. Fumes are also produced by the heating of any metal above its melting point (Seeger, p. 41).

Because of the number of chemicals involved, and the variety of possible mixtures, identifying a few general guidelines to reduce hazards is not really possible. Ceramics teachers, therefore, have a special obligation to keep up with the technical literature relating to safety. They should continually question manufacturers about health and safety hazards related to their products. Some important questions are:

- What is the exact nature of the chemical changes caused by firing glaze substances? What fumes are likely to be released and how can protection from the most hazardous be provided? Are there chemicals which must not be mixed because of a synergistic effect in the firing?
- What is the best location for the specific kiln(s) in use? If they are inside the building, what is the volume of air (cfm) necessary to insure fumes are carried off through a canopy hood? How far should a kiln be located from a flammable wall surface?
- What is the maintenance schedule to be followed for each specific kiln type and kiln part? Who is qualified to carry out maintenance? Do the kilns require inspection by a fire marshal? What type of periodic inspections should be done and by whom?
- What safety controls are available for each kiln to prevent overfiring or missed shutoff times?

It is reasonable to expect the manufacturer or the distributor of materials and equipment to give answers to these questions; if they expect to continue to supply products to schools, they must accept the responsibility of working with teachers to develop the most hazard-free conditions.

Clay is a wonderfully creative medium in which to work and there is no reason for conditions to exist which make it an unsafe medium if the general precautions outlined here are followed. The full-time or specialist ceramics teacher, who is probably also a serious potter, will need to constantly search for information from sources such as NIOSH, OSHA, and the Center for Occupational Hazards. NIOSH and OSHA are agencies of the Department of Labor and can be contacted for information through the regional offices of that department. COH is a private non-profit organization and is located at 5 Beekman Street, New York, NY, 10038.

PHOTOGRAPHY

Recently, photography has become an increasingly important part of many art programs. Once the high school darkroom was under the control of the English department and used only for developing the pictures used in the school annual. Now the darkroom is often a facility central to the entire art program. With the production of new and relatively inexpensive equipment, including good quality 35 mm cameras, many students will have formal training in photography in the seventh grade or earlier. Pinhole cameras and film developing are not uncommon experiences even in the third grade.

Of all processes, photography is the most dependent on chemicals. It is, in fact, totally a process of chemical manipulation, from the first exposure of the film to the printing of the picture. Consequently teachers who direct students in photo work should know, for example, which chemicals may cause some health problems, which should not be used, which can be mixed together safely and which should not be allowed to stand in a bath. This information is essential to students learning photo processes, so if they continue to do photo work in their own darkrooms at home, they will not be putting themselves and others in jeopardy.

Unfortunately, most teachers know little about the chemicals they are using in photography. Labels will usually identify the chemical contents (and many include valuable warning information), but they are helpful only if the teacher already understands about the chemicals. Nevertheless, as discussed earlier, label information is extremely important in explaining as much as possible about the contents so appropriate decisions can be made. The *Compact Lab Index* (Pittaro, 1977) provides valuable data on precautions to be taken in photo processing. It is an extremely useful guide to the correct methods of mixing chemicals and temperature control requirements to achieve good results under safe conditions.

Fundamentally, the photo teacher has the responsibility to know: which chemicals should be avoided and which photo processes should not be done in a school setting; ventilation requirements for the darkroom; and the necessary precautions for handling any chemicals.

Chemicals and Processes to Avoid

Figure 12 lists several chemicals which should be avoided because they are highly toxic, difficult to handle safely and are not essential to quality photo experience for students. In most cases, these chemicals will not be found in school programs, but the photo instructor should double-check to be sure and confirm that these chemicals are not part of any regularly used compounds. In addition to these specific chemicals, several photo processes depend on chemicals too hazardous for use in a typical school program. These processes are identified in Figure 13. There may be some schools with very advanced photo courses where some of the processes (e.g., color) may be appropriate. But these are exceptional instances and the teacher has a special obligation to understand all of the hazards and ways of controlling them. An excellent source of complete and highly professional information on photo hazards is available in *Overexposure: Health Hazards in Photography* (Shaw, 1983). This should be used as a specific guide in solving photo program hazard problems.

Perhaps the best general advice is that both student and teacher always have the choice of avoiding especially hazardous chemicals or processes. For example, if a student has a thin negative which has to be "built up" by a chemical intensifier, the choice *should* be to reshoot the picture. Only rarely will the situation warrant this sort of chemical manipulation. Then, a professional photographer should do the work.

Darkroom Ventilation

Professional photographers recommend general ventilation with ten air changes per hour for the darkroom. To dilute the contamination from

TOXIC CHEMICALS TO BE AVOIDED IN THE SCHOOL PHOTO PROGRAM[1,2]

Chemical	Hazard
Developers	

Catechin
  catechol
  pyrocatechol
  o-dihydroxybenzene
	Difficulty in breathing; cyanosis, liver-kidney damage; ingestion may be fatal.

Pyrogallic acid pyrogallol	Cyanosis, anemia, liver-kidney damage; ingestion can be fatal.
Diaminophenol hydrochloride	Severe skin irritation, bronchial asthma, gastritis, convulsions, coma.
Intensifiers	
Mercuric chloride	Chronic mercury poisoning.
Mercuric iodide	Chronic mercury poisoning.
Potassium cyanide	Rashes, chemical asphyxia; ingestion can be fatal.
Uranium nitrate	Skin corrosion, liver-kidney damage; radioactive.
Toner	
Thiourea	Causes cancer in rats; suspected carcinogen.
Miscellaneous	
Formaldehyde	Sensitizer causing respiratory and skin allergies; suspected carcinogen.
Freons (fluorocarbons)	Respiratory irritations; heating may produce poison gases.

1. Seeger, *A Photographer's Guide to the Safe Use of Materials,* pp. 29–40.
2. McCann, *Artist Beware,* pp. 310–324.

Figure 12.

PHOTO PROCESSES TO BE AVOIDED
IN THE SCHOOLS[1,2]

Teachers must individually make decisions concerning these processes, but
their use is not recommended because the potential hazards are so serious
that controlling them is expensive. If a teacher has a special interest in
one of these processes, it is suggested that after becoming fully aware of
the potential hazards, the use of the process be kept for the teacher's own
personal creative work and not attempted with students.

Process	Rationale for Avoidance
Color processing:	Many of the chemicals used in color processing are highly toxic and require local exhaust and very careful control methods. It is a complex, difficult process and should only be undertaken in the most advanced classes under the direction of extremely well qualified instructors.
Cibachrome:	Highly toxic chemicals used in this process are suspected especially of affecting the female reproductive system, possibly resulting in birth defects and miscarriages.
Gum printing:	Requires local ventilation; dust masks must be worn when using powders. Results probably do not warrant the precautions necessary.
Cyanotype:	Exposure by carbon arc light on potassium ferricyanide can release hydrogen cyanide gas. Eyes and skin are especially sensitive to UV radiation. Can be done safely if exposure is by sunlight and water is used for developing.
Daguerreotype:	Exposure to highly toxic mercury vapor is possible; educational results do not seem to warrant the risk.

Figure 13.

1. Seeger, *A Photographer's Guide to the Safe Use of Materials.*
2. McCann, *Artist Beware.*

chemicals normally in use, fresh air must be brought into the room to replace the old air ten times during every hour. Some ventilation experts feel this "rule of thumb" is inappropriate in many uses (Hemeon, 1963) and is, in any case, a difficult concept for a teacher to use meaningfully. Three steps should be taken in determining what constitutes effective ventilation. First, gather all possible information about the chemicals used in the darkroom, including the amount to be used at any one time. Second, collect information on appropriate ventilation systems and recommended standards from available sources (Shaw, pp. 66–74; Clark, et al; ACGIH Ventilation Manual). Third, take that information to the school's personnel responsible for designing and maintaining school ventilation systems. Get that person to apply the information to your specific room. This is not a job for the teacher alone. A conscientious teacher should know the chemicals, the number of student stations and the size of the space. Calculating adequate air exchange and designing the system is a task for people expert in doing that.

Local exhaust configurations will probably not be necessary if the chemicals and processes identified in Figures 12 and 13 are not used. Teachers who, for reasons of personal interest or experience, want the students to work with these processes must acknowledge the need for expensive local exhaust equipment which, at best, will only reduce and not control the hazards. The question, of course, is whether those processes have sufficient educational value to the students to justify this cost.

Handling the Chemicals

Several simple rules should govern the handling of chemicals in photo processing:

- Wear gloves. Regular household gloves are not adequate protection from the chemicals, so check with chemical suppliers to get recommendations for the most effective type. Neoprene or neoprene-latex gloves will probably be appropriate in most cases, but do not guess.
- Wash gloves, inside and out, after use and thoroughly wash hands as well.
- If any skin irritation should result from wearing gloves, use tongs instead, but be sure to keep hands out of the chemicals, especially

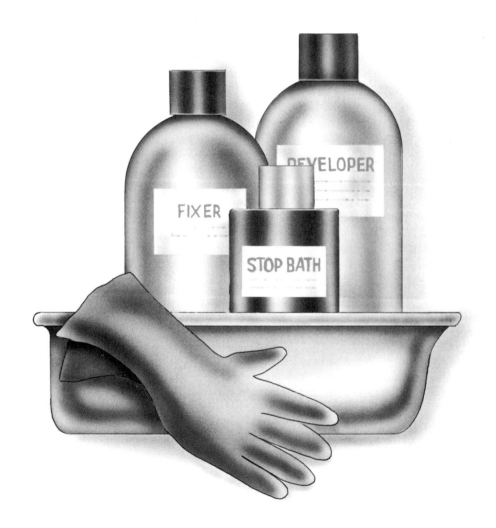

developers. "Most developing baths can be highly hazardous to the skin, particularly with continued use because the effects on the skin can be cumulative" (Seeger, 1983, p. 30).

- Have a skin and eye wash facility available in the darkroom to allow immediate flushing of chemical splashes.
- Do not heat chemicals to speed their action. Heating usually causes erratic results and most often produces bad negatives or prints anyway; heating can also produce toxic chemical fumes.
- Keep all chemical baths covered when not in use so the fumes caused by evaporation are reduced as much as possible.
- Do not allow sodium thiosulphate (fixer) to become old, since it may decompose to produce sulfur dioxide. Do not heat it, and always keep it covered when not in use.
- Clean up spills so they do not dry and form dust that can contaminate the air.

In general any process as popular and as chemically intensive as photography requires special attention to its hazards. Many of these students will not have had any previous art experience, and some will have no subsequent classes in art, so their entire attitude about what constitutes safe practices in art will depend on what goes on in photography. It is also probable that many of those who take photography will continue to work with it in and out of school settings. They need to be carefully instructed in the requirements for setting up a safe home darkroom. For these reasons, photo teachers bear a heavy responsibility in providing instruction and information that is complete and accurate. The school photo program should exemplify a safe and hazard-controlled operation.

SCULPTURE

All three dimensional activities are likely to be classified as sculpture. This can mean anything from a simple cut and folded paper form to a cast object involving modeling, mold making, metal heating and pouring, grinding, polishing and adding patina. Except that the objects created in each case occupy three dimensions, and are viewed as such, they have little in common.

The sculpture processes normally seen in the elementary school do not go much beyond various paper or cardboard constructions fastened with glue and staples, papier-mâché, simple wood constructions, clay and perhaps wire worked in combination with scrap materials. There are of course some hazards involved with each of these, such as the use of certain adhesives, cutting tools, and the problems of any clay activities. These hazards have already been discussed in earlier chapters. The sculpture activities of concern here are those likely to be done in the junior and senior high school. These involve more advanced methods and materials.

Realistically, there are many sculpture processes well within the capabilities of secondary level students which are almost never done because of the cost and complexity of materials and equipment. Metal casting foundries, for example, rarely exist in high school art areas. Similarly, the equipment for vaccum forming plastics might be available to high school students but only in exceptional settings. Where these processes exist, the teachers must demonstrate extreme concern for the health and safety of the students. These teachers must be familiar with the highly technical information specifically directed to sculpture with those media (McCann, 1979; Siedlecki, 1972).

Similarly, using plastics to make sculpture has dropped significantly in popularity and frequency in recent years, probably in part because the health hazards of the various epoxies and resins have become better known. Many of the exciting visual possibilities these materials once seemed to have, no longer are so attractive to artists, students or teachers. Although plastics in many forms continue to have widespread commercial application, only a few professional artists, and rarely junior or senior high school students, use them.

There is actually little to recommend plastics as a sculptural medium in the secondary schools. It should be used only in special circumstances and directed by artists knowledgeable in the health hazards. Moreover, any process involving heating or dissolving plastics for sculptural constructions should absolutely not be done in the elementary or junior high school levels. The risks are too great, and the possibilities of controlling them too unrealistic.

Wood Carving and Construction

These involve hand or power cutting tools which have been discussed in earlier sections of this book. In addition, however, it is important to emphasize the necessity of wearing eye protection and being sure work is done in a location where non-involved students will not be injured by flying chips or errant pieces of wood. Sanding and polishing wood are not particularly hazardous activities unless power equipment is used improperly. Belt or orbital sanders are relatively easy to control and should cause little difficulty, although large floor models sometimes move at a speed which can pull a piece of wood away from an inattentive student. All tools should be equipped with proper guards. Power sawing and sanding produce significant quantities of wood dust, much of which is suspended in the air for some period of time. Fixed sanding equipment or saws should be fitted with vacuum dust collecting systems, and students should wear appropriate dust masks if there is extensive wood working going on. Typically there will not be enough dust in an art classroom for this to be a serious problem, but an aware teacher will take the proper precautions, should dusty conditions prevail.

Finishing materials used with wood primarily involve solvents, which have already been discussed, and since the adhesive most often used in attaching pieces is non-toxic white plastic glue, few problems exist in this area.

Metal Forming—Welding

In some schools, metal sculpture has grown in popularity and welding is not an uncommon practice. Although most metal work occurs in an industrial arts shop rather than the artroom, some aspects of metal forming and joining may be found there. The major hazards in working with metal involve cutting, either with hand-held metal snips or large guillotine-type cutting presses. Under no circumstances should the latter be used without extensive training and careful supervison. In fact, where work of this scale is undertaken, an especially thorough skill testing program should exist.

Welding is a similar case. The most common types of welding include oxygen-acetylene, arc welding and brazing. Of these, arc welding is probably the least likely to be found in any secondary school art program. Teachers whose students arc-weld should consult, as a minimum, publications such as *Welding Safety* (NIOSH, 1977) or the *Accident Prevention Manual for Industrial Operations* (McElroy, 1969). Welding in any of its forms, however, is a very specialized task and requires a fully trained and experienced teacher to prevent accidents. Welding should not be considered a process students can pursue "creatively" without a complete and thorough grounding in correct procedures. The following rules should be considered minimum guidelines for safe welding activities:

- Read and follow all warning labels.
- Always check to be sure equipment is in good working order.
- Acetylene and oxygen tanks must always be chained to a wall or to a substantial portable cart to insure they do not fall over and damage gauges or fittings.
- Use correct protective equipment (masks, clothing and gloves).
- Work inside only if there is an effective ventilation system and then stand so as to avoid breathing any of the fumes rising from the work. If working outside, be sure fumes blow away from other persons and building openings.
- Be very careful of fire. Keep all flammable materials well away from the work area and be sure to have an appropriate fire extinguisher within easy reach.

Welding and brazing produce various air contaminants from the rods and the metals being joined as well as from coatings or painted surfaces which produce fumes when heated. Most of these fumes are difficult to identify, and they should all be assumed to be harmful and so require proper ventilation.

Generally, there are an almost unlimited number of materials and processes that can be used to make sculpture. The simplest of these usually involve no unexpected hazards. However, the more complex processes, such as metal forming and casting or work in plastics, are not ones which should be undertaken in most school art programs. The teacher must not only be skilled in the processes to teach them effectively, but fully aware of the health and safety hazards they create. These problems will not be easy or inexpensive to solve, and a careful evaluation of the educational and aesthetic goals of the art program should be made to determine the importance of such activities in the program.

JEWELRYMAKING

Complex manipulation of materials and tools even at elementary levels demands careful attention to potential hazards in jewelrymaking. Most teachers recognize that the cutting, filing, casting, soldering or polishing inherent in this craft have the potential for causing a variety of injuries. Consequently safety is a normal part of instructional procedures in jewelrymaking. Wearing goggles during grinding and polishing is probably the most obvious protection. If teachers follow normal practices they will absolutely require eye protection for even brief periods. More detailed discussion of eye protection is found in Chapter Three.

In addition to eye protection, sufficient ventilation is necessary to remove fumes and fine dust particles from many steps in the process. For example, in mixing the dry powder to make an investment mold for lost wax casting, ventilation is needed to protect the student from inhaling the dust which may contain up to 30 percent silica, a long-term cause of silicosis. Dust is also a problem when breaking up investment molds. Proper ventilation also insures that fumes from molten metals are not inhaled. If brass or bronze are being cast, there will be trace amounts of beryllium and arsenic in these copper alloys, and their effects can be very serious. Furnaces used for burn-out of the wax in this process also must be located near effective ventilation.

Local ventilation will also protect students from soldering fumes created by the materials used for flux: cadmium, fluorides, and perhaps lead. Intense exposure to these can be dangerous, but if the fumes are drawn away by an effective air movement system, the dangers are relatively slight.

For many years, jewelry studios used asbestos blocks or boards as heat resistant surfaces on which to solder. Few teachers cannot know the dangers of asbestos fibers which can often be broken loose from these objects. Since no amount of exposure to asbestos fibers is considered acceptable, immediately and correctly dispose of any such blocks or boards. Be sure to check with the school administration about how this can most safely be done; schools do not take student exposure to asbestos lightly.

Several general observations can be made about how to eliminate or control jewelry hazards.

- Be sure all machine guards are in place and in use on any grinding or polishing tools in the room.
- Clearly instruct students on how to cut and saw metal or wire. Proper metal snips or coping saws should be used; vises or clamps should hold metal in place during the cutting, and safety glasses

or goggles should be used. Be sure to file rough metal edges to reduce cuts or scratches.

- Heat metal only where local ventilation is available. In soldering or melting metals for casting, fumes should be drawn away from the student; it may be necessary to have individual elephant trunk hoods at work stations to insure full protection.
- Wear eye protection and work only in an area with good general ventilation when polishing; be sure long hair and sleeves are securely tied back to prevent tangling in the polishing wheel.
- Handle acids used in the pickling process (nitric, sulphuric, sodium bisulfate) with great care. Wear gloves, always add acid to water in mixing the solution, and keep acid baths covered when not in use. When the acids should be disposed of, be sure to follow methods prescribed for the school—do not simply pour the diluted solution down the drain. If there is no disposal policy, request that school officials find out how it should be done so city water treatment facilities are not damaged. Pickling acids need local exhaust ventilation.
- Keep work areas clean and dust-free.
- Periodically check torches and all hoses to be sure they are in good condition and do not leak.
- Use only cadmium-free silver solders and fluoride-free fluxes.
- Use lead-free enamels.
- Develop rules to be followed in the use of protective equipment.

Perhaps the best way to introduce jewelrymaking to students is to have them design and work with very simple materials such as string, yarn, leather thongs and found objects which can be manipulated into body adornment. As they develop a sense of how materials can work together, wire and plastic can be explored. When they are ready to try their ideas entirely in metals, they will then have a good sense about jewelry design and will find the safety requirements easier to manage. If students understand design concepts, they will have far less trouble in understanding and accepting health and safety precautions.

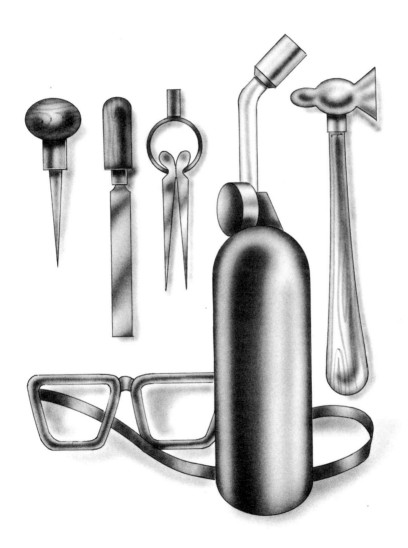

Part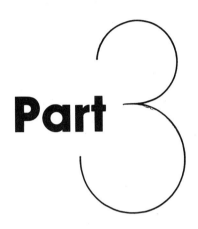

CURRICULUM
AND LEGAL
CONCERNS

8

Curriculum and Safety

SCHOOL AND COMMUNITY ACTION

The art teacher's time should be spent teaching art under healthy and safe conditions which enhance student learning. The role of the administration is to efficiently allocate the available physical environment and fiscal resources to accomplish that goal. As always, cooperation between teacher and administration is essential to bring about needed improvements.

Teachers must realize that their role is not, however, limited to working with the students in the classroom. They must make a concerted effort to keep the administration informed of the problems, needs and proposals for improving artroom health and safety conditions. In the past, art supervisors and program coordinators played a large role in planning program changes and choosing materials and equipment. Much could be left to the "central office." In most schools, that centralization no longer exists, and these tasks fall upon the individual teacher and principal. While many lament the loss of a person in the district who can organize and standardize such matters, teachers have to recognize the role is now theirs and accept the responsibility for it.

No one can tell a teacher what type of health and safety advocacy will work best with a specific principal. Administrative style and personality vary greatly, and the teacher's ability to "read" that style and personality is fundamental to any effort to gain support. There are some basic actions which may be effective in achieving results:

- Organize a health and safety program including a student committee, procedures for the inventory and investigation of all art materials, specific housekeeping practices to reduce hazards, a procedure for testing student competency and a complete record file.
- Assess the art program to identify hazardous activities and develop either plans to cope with the hazards or to replace the activity with one of equal value.
- Keep the principal fully informed of plans, actions and accomplishments.
- Request expert advice on technical matters. Don't call in the fire marshal without the principal's knowledge, but be aware that specialized answers can come only from specialists.
- Involve other teachers and school and community personnel in the health and safety program.
- Seek advice from the school nurse.

Effective health and safety program work will benefit from involving people outside the art program. It gives them the opportunity to share special knowledge and skills with the students and to feel they are making an important contribution to the schools. It is also possible that this involvement will enlist support not only of a health and safety effort but of the role of art in the school curriculum.

PROGRAM PLANNING

The root of any art hazard lies in the art program itself. It is the selection of components which determine materials and processes, which in turn affect the nature of any hazards. Art programs develop as they do for a number of reasons, often having little to do with the students' specific needs.

Some art programs result from inertia. The teacher inherited a closet full of supplies which had to be used up, and once the sequence of projects got started, it was too much trouble to change.

Some art programs result from popularity. Unless certain courses are offered, enrollment will drop, and the art program will be eliminated.

Some art programs aren't really programs at all but the product of expedience. They comprise projects that caught the teacher's fancy, were interesting to the kids or satisfied the need for some holiday. These projects only serve to keep the kids busy and may have nothing to do with one another and little to do with learning about art.

And some art programs are a response to pressure — the expectations of the parents, the principal or a curriculum guide.

Most art programs are a mixture of all the above, and, if the mix is a sensitive one, they may be very good. There is certainly nothing wrong with meeting student interests or parent expectations, but teachers must plan programs carefully. If there are health or safety hazards involved, they must weigh the problem against the benefits. Is it an activity essential to the goals of both the program and the school?

Careful program planning is thus critically important in determining what hazards must be surmounted. Good planning also makes it infinitely easier to justify any special costs in doing so. A teacher who rationally demonstrates that an activity is absolutely essential will effectively rally support for safety expenditures.

PROPOSING CHANGES: STRATEGY

Do the easy things first. This will initiate a strategy to bring about a healthy and safe artroom environment. For example, if ventilation is thought to be the most serious problem in a particular artroom, demanding a ventilation system be installed immediately may not be the best tactic. First remedy the secondary factors which contribute to the ventilation problem. Because ventilation systems are usually expensive, such requests will hold more weight if all other possible actions have been taken to reduce the problem of poor air quality. Demonstrating a commitment to alleviating the problem on all fronts will help convince the administration that a new ventilation system is a necessity. But remember, no ventilation system can blow away problems that originate in program planning or teacher practices which are inherently indifferent to the creation of hazards.

Each school district has a somewhat different method for instituting changes in such things as room assignment, allocating space for storage and setting capital improvement priorities. Art teachers must work within the normal channels to bring about their requests. An artroom may need more storage, a separate room for clay mixing, local ventilation for kilns, or significant replacement or addition of tools and equipment. Such projects always compete for dollars with such proposals as improvements to the cafeteria, installation of handicapped facilities, repair of furnaces, replacement of broken windows or a gymnasium floor and landscaping for the school grounds. It is formidable competition. To compete successfully, consider the following:

- Learn the system. Find out what things influence decision-making. Is it cost, enrollment figures, pressure from outside groups or a bias to some areas as opposed to others? Without understanding both the system and the politics behind it, proposals will have only a slim chance.
- What are upward limits for any single project? Can projects be split into phases and receive a funding commitment for a two- or three-year period?
- What external support would be helpful? Would it harm the proposal's chances to seek PTA or other outside group aid in either advocating or fund raising?
- Who are the people most influential in making the decision, and how can they be convinced of the proposal's importance?

There is no sure way to succeed in funding a health and safety proposal. Even in the best of economic circumstances, correcting hazards in an artroom is never a sure thing. There is, however, no substitute for a meticulously prepared plan: the successful teachers will have done their homework thoroughly. Art programs usually don't have the luxury of the almost automatic support often given science or athletic activities, so the task will not be easy.

Two additional points should be made concerning strategy: first, do not use scare tactics, and second, don't provide the solutions for the problems.

If the problems are presented in a strident and threatening manner, the art program will very likely suffer. Claiming that the problems can only be solved with large quantities of money may only convince administrators it isn't worth the cost.

Providing solutions to the problems should be left to experts; teachers should only compile the data about the use of problem materials used and about the activities that take place. Some teachers may be very well informed about hazards, but, nonetheless, do not have the technical knowledge to correct them. Moreover, should a teacher-designed system go wrong, there usually is no possibility for further corrections. Recognizing the problem and designing the solution are different jobs, and the wise teacher will not confuse them.

SUBSTITUTING MATERIALS AND PROCEDURES

The substitution of non-toxic for toxic materials has already been emphasized as an important way to control hazards. What has not been said, however, is that substitution of materials is not free, nor is it a step that can usually be taken quickly or easily. The substitution may involve changing activities or changing the kind of materials used within an activity. In any case, the changeover requires the selection and ordering of safer materials that may be more expensive, and these will take time to be ordered and delivered. Unless the decision to change materials is made at exactly the right time in the budgetary cycle, it may be as much a year or longer before the substitute supplies arrive in the artroom. It may also be difficult and time-consuming to find appropriate substitutes.

This is not intended to discourage substitution practices, but rather emphasize the need to plan ahead. How can the changes be made as expeditiously as possible?

The key is the person responsible for ordering supplies for the school district. It may be necessary to discuss procedure with the school principal, but usually the district purchasing agent (who in some cases may be the school principal) will cooperate to insure that the new materials are safer than the old ones and explain how specifications must be written to receive what is expected.

Whether to continue using unlabeled materials or to substitute other, perhaps less satisfactory materials is a difficult decision, and the purchasing agent can help. Ask him or her to request a Material Safety Data Sheet from the manufacturer to get toxicity information (Figure 14). This document describes the potential hazards of materials and should be supplied on request. If this information is not forthcoming, let that be a signal to avoid that particular material and possibly to consider making no further orders from that manufacturer. Art materials manufacturers have a special

U.S. DEPARTMENT OF LABOR Occupational Safety and Health Administration	Form Approved OMB No. 44-R1387

MATERIAL SAFETY DATA SHEET

Required under USDL Safety and Health Regulations for Ship Repairing,
Shipbuilding, and Shipbreaking (29 CFR 1915, 1916, 1917)

SECTION I

MANUFACTURER'S NAME	EMERGENCY TELEPHONE NO.
ADDRESS *(Number, Street, City, State, and ZIP Code)*	
CHEMICAL NAME AND SYNONYMS	TRADE NAME AND SYNONYMS
CHEMICAL FAMILY	FORMULA

SECTION II - HAZARDOUS INGREDIENTS

PAINTS, PRESERVATIVES, & SOLVENTS	%	TLV (Units)	ALLOYS AND METALLIC COATINGS	%	TLV (Units)
PIGMENTS			BASE METAL		
CATALYST			ALLOYS		
VEHICLE			METALLIC COATINGS		
SOLVENTS			FILLER METAL PLUS COATING OR CORE FLUX		
ADDITIVES			OTHERS		
OTHERS					

HAZARDOUS MIXTURES OF OTHER LIQUIDS, SOLIDS, OR GASES	%	TLV (Units)

SECTION III - PHYSICAL DATA

BOILING POINT (°F.)		SPECIFIC GRAVITY (H$_2$O=1)	
VAPOR PRESSURE (mm Hg.)		PERCENT, VOLATILE BY VOLUME (%)	
VAPOR DENSITY (AIR=1)		EVAPORATION RATE (_____ =1)	
SOLUBILITY IN WATER			
APPEARANCE AND ODOR			

SECTION IV - FIRE AND EXPLOSION HAZARD DATA

FLASH POINT (Method used)	FLAMMABLE LIMITS	Lel	Uel
EXTINGUISHING MEDIA			
SPECIAL FIRE FIGHTING PROCEDURES			
UNUSUAL FIRE AND EXPLOSION HAZARDS			

Figure 14.

obligation to be open with teachers who are selecting materials to be used by young people. If they refuse to accept that responsibility, schools should not buy their products. If a sense of moral obligation doesn't move the manufacturer, perhaps the economic pressure will.

EXTREME SOLUTIONS

Sometimes all efforts fail to correct a hazard: the substitution of activities or materials may not be desirable; cleaning the artroom does not accomplish the expected effects; there are no funds to make physical improvements or to remodel the existing room; perhaps the classes are just too large for the space. Every teacher must face the possibility that sometimes the hazards cannot be eliminated by these means.

In this situation, there are still two possible courses of action: either totally change the program, or change either the location of the artroom or the location of the hazardous activities. In all probability moving will be the best choice.

Getting support to move may not be difficult if the case is well made. The teacher must of course document the need, suggest new locations and outline the benefits and costs of such a move. However, the purpose of such a move must not be to increase space or improve conditions other than those related to the problem.

9

Legal Liability

LEGAL IMPLICATIONS OF ARTROOM HAZARDS

Genuine concern for students should be sufficient motivation for teachers to make health and safety an integral part of their art programs. But the possibility of becoming a defendant in a law suit may be needed to move some teachers to recognize their obligations to students. In a society which has increasingly turned to the courts to solve problems, law suits are an ever-present reality for teachers. Judgments in the hundreds of thousands of dollars are common in damage actions, and the number of times a teacher is the defendant in such cases can be expected to increase in the future.

Art teachers need to be aware of their vulnerability to legal action and of steps they should take to protect themselves. Stated in another way, "Because of the age, maturity, and experience limitations of most students, and because teachers stand *in loco parentis* (in the place of a parent), schools are expected to provide a safe environment and establish reasonable behavior for the protection of students" (Florio, 1979, p. 222).

Negligence is the charge most likely to be brought against an art teacher. In cases where students were injured in the artroom, the teacher has often been sued for negligence on the grounds that the injury wouldn't have occurred had there been proper instruction and supervision: the teacher should therefore be liable for damages. In general, there are several defenses a teacher can use in court. But no examples in school law literature specifically refer to art teachers or to injuries occurring in artrooms. Moreover, cases in which the damages were sought for negligence resulting in illness rather than injury are likewise not mentioned. There is little comfort for the art teacher in this. Everyone should take extra precautions because precedents do not seem to exist, and someone may be seeking them.

However, "it must be emphasized that a teacher is not liable for personal damages every time a student under the teacher's supervision is injured in an accident " (Flygare, 1976, p. 42). It is important to know under what circumstances the teacher can be held liable. An affirmative answer to each of the following four questions indicates liability:

1. Did the defendant have a duty or responsibility to the plaintiff? Was there an obligation to protect the plaintiff against unreasonable risk of harm?
2. Was there a failure to conform to the required standard of care owed the plaintiff? This question establishes the existence of negligence, which is the dominant principle of tort law.
3. Was there a causal connection between failure to provide adequate care and resulting injury (proximate cause)?
4. Did an actual loss or damage result from the commission or omission of an action by the defendant? (Prosser, 1971, quoted in Florio, et al., 1979, p. 220.)

The teacher needs to relate each of these four questions to the artroom situation and take steps to be sure the answers are negative. In this way, protection against tort action should be assured so far as is now known.

DUTY OR RESPONSIBILITY

There are three questions about duty or responsibility that must be established by the injured person:

1. That the defendant had a duty to protect the injured person.
2. That the defendant failed to do that.
3. That the failure was the proximate cause (a substantial factor) of the injury (Peterson, 1978, p. 252).

Duty involves the issue of "standard of care," and it has been interpreted that teachers "are held to be a higher standard of care than the ordinary man on the street. The teacher or administrator is under the duty to possess more than the 'ordinary' amount of intelligence in relation to students and their care" (Gatti, 1975, p. 213).

The required standard of care may be considered less for high school students than for elementary school students because of differences in age and maturity. The actual determination of this difference is a matter for a jury to decide as a "question of fact."

Proximate cause means that the injury must have been "proximately caused" by an act or there is no liability (Gatti, p. 178). For example, if the teacher omitted some instruction, and the injury would not have occurred had the instruction been given, then it was "proximately caused" by that failure and there has been negligence on the part of the teacher. It becomes especially important, therefore, for the teacher not to assume the students are familiar with any activity or tool use. Always give instructions pertaining to them. The question that will be asked in court is, "Did the injury occur because of something the teacher did or *did not* do?" For a teacher to be held blameless, it cannot be found that something was overlooked when the students were given instructions for their work.

FORESEEABILITY AND TEACHER-MADE RULES

"When a teacher or administrator foresees or reasonably could foresee that an injury might occur if a particular condition is not corrected or preventative action is not taken, he or she has a duty to do something about it prior to the injury occurring. If he or she does not, liability may be imposed for negligence" (Gatti, p. 133). The "reasonable and prudent" teacher must insure that the problems are corrected before injury or illness occurs and establish rules about student conduct where a problem situation exists. If the condition cannot be corrected by the teacher, a formal written request to have it done should be made to the school administrator immediately with a copy kept for the teacher's own records.

Teachers have the right, as well as responsibility, to make rules enforcing safe procedures. To be legally binding, the rules must be written, should be clearly understandable and concise, must be communicated to the students and must be enforced. "Many teachers are sued and held liable for simply not having enforced rules regarding health and safety of their students . . . Remember, the rules must be reasonable, lawful, and cannot conflict with the student's constitutional rights" (Gatti, p. 226).

CONTRIBUTORY NEGLIGENCE AND ASSUMPTION OF RISK

If a student is injured by behaving in a manner that jeopardizes his or her own safety, that behavior may be defined as contributory negligence. If a student is guilty of contributory negligence, no damages can be recovered. But the burden of proving that negligence is on the defendant (in this case, the teacher), who must show that the student's behavior in part caused the injury. In this type of defense, it must be determined whether the student, given his or her age, could be expected to understand the nature and extent of the danger. If the student could not be expected to know, then the behavior would not be considered contributory.

Assumption of risk is a legal defense based on the contention that the student assumed the risk of injury by participating in the activity. But "an essential requisite to invoking the assumption of risk doctrine is that there be not only knowledge of a physical defect in the premises, but also appreciation of the danger produced by the physical defect" (Peterson, p. 256). In respect to the artroom environment, this defense depends heavily on whether the student was properly instructed about the hazards involved in the activity, and whether the student actually had that knowledge.

INTERVENING ACTS

If a teacher actually has not fulfilled his or her responsibilities in exercising the proper care, damages would still probably not be assessed in a negligence case if some intervening act was found to be the proximate cause of the injury. "In some instances an intervening event, such as the negligence of a third party, has relieved school personnel of liability" (McCarthy, 1981, p. 176). However, a judgment might still be rendered against the teacher in such a case if there is reason to believe the teacher should have anticipated and prevented that intervening act.

Suppose, for example, a teacher has failed to provide careful instructions and warned about the dangers in using a paper cutter. In a later classroom incident, a student loses a finger directly as the result of careless behavior of another student at the paper cutter. Although the second student's action would be an intervening act, there may be reason to believe the teacher is still liable if it can be shown that teachers should always anticipate problems when two students use the cutter at one time. Obviously, hoping there may be an intervening act should hardly be an excuse for inadequate initial instruction, and teachers should always give appropriate instruction and carefully monitor the behavior of the students at all times.

WAIVER OF LIABILITY— PERMISSION SLIPS

It is common belief that to have a parent sign a permission slip for a student activity constitutes a waiver of the teacher's liability in the event of student injury or illness during that activity. However, "negligence is not among the risks accepted by parents on behalf of their children" (Florio, p. 224), and a permission slip simply indicates the parents are aware their child is participating in the activity. The principal value of such a slip is that if an injury does occur, and there has been no teacher negligence, it can be used as a defense against any charges by the parents that the activity was not one in which the child should have participated. If, however, negligence can be proved, the teacher is still liable for damages regardless of there being a signed permission slip.

PROVIDING MEDICAL ASSISTANCE

Giving medical assistance may result in litigation if it is not deemed reasonable and prudent under the circumstances. In an emergency, the teacher is expected to provide first aid if no medical personnel are available or if the injury is such that attention cannot wait the arrival of a nurse or doctor. But a person acting in an emergency "cannot be held to the same standard of care as one who has had time to reflect. Even if it later appears that the defendant made a decision which no reasonable person could possibly have made after careful deliberation, there is no negligence" (Prosser quoted in Florio, p. 223). Not to give any treatment in an emergency situation, however, is considered negligent, but any treatment must not cause the condition to become worse. If that should happen, the teacher might be held liable for causing a more severe injury than was originally incurred.

AVOIDING LITIGATION

There are several actions teachers can take to reduce the chance of a law suit charging negligence. The best, of course, is "the prevention of injury through competent instruction and adequate supervision" (Florio, p. 225). However, several other actions are of equal importance:

- Insure that dangerous conditions have been eliminated.
  1. Maintain the room in a safe manner with equipment properly located for safe use and be sure that hazards arising from the room itself are identified and eliminated.
  2. Keep all equipment in good working order: sharp cutting edges, electrical cords in good condition, proper kinds of protective gear available.
  3. Store materials and tools in appropriate containers and/or cabinets and clearly identify the contents.
- Establish rules of behavior and enforce them.
  1. Make sure rules are clear, concise and understood.
  2. Put rules in writing and either distribute them to the students or, if appropriate, post them in the area where the activities they govern take place.
  3. Require responsible behavior. Do not allow immature actions to go unchecked, and be sure all offenders are disciplined.
- Formally test students' understanding of correct procedures.
  1. Be sure students are carefully instructed in the correct use of all materials and equipment.
  2. Develop and use tests to verify students have both knowledge and skills to participate in art activities. (See Figures 15 and 16 for test examples.)

SAMPLE COMPETENCY ESSAY TEST

Competency Test   Name: _____

* Electric Kiln Operation *   Date: _____

                                     Class: _____

                                     Teacher: _____

1. Describe each step that must be taken to safely bring the kiln to full firing temperature once it has been loaded. Be very precise in your answer.

   a.

   b.

   c.

   d.

2. How long must a kiln cool before the lid may safely be opened?

3. What kind and amount of room ventilation is required when an electric kiln is being fired?

4. What specific precautions must be taken in checking cones during kiln firing?

5. (Optional, if appropriate.) Describe the steps that must be taken to activate the automatic electric kiln control equipment.

Figure 15.

This example should be modified to fit specific settings, expected student responsibilities, and the type of equipment used.

SAMPLE COMPETENCY TEST — MULTIPLE CHOICE AND OBSERVATION

Competency Test

* Linoleum Printmaking Tools *

Name: _____

Date: _____

TEACHER OBSERVATION OF STUDENT SKILLS (INITIAL APPROVAL) _____	Class: _____
	Teacher: _____

Check as many answers as you believe are correct.

1. Linoleum blocks are only to be cut using what tool?

    a. Paring knife _____
    b. Linoleum knives _____
    c. Linoleum cutting tools _____
    d. Razor blade _____

2. A bench hook is used for what purpose in linoleum block printing?

    a. To hang coats on benches _____
    b. To support the block while cutting _____
    c. To print the block _____
    d. To hook the linoleum to the bench _____

3. How can you tell when a cutting blade is too dull to use safely?

    a. It slips across the block without cutting _____
    b. It doesn't cut the block easily _____
    c. It takes on a dull color _____
    d. It has been discarded by someone else _____

4. If it is necessary to hold the linoleum block with your hand, how should it be held?

    a. In front of the cutting tool _____
    b. Between the cutting tool and your body _____
    c. Away from the path of the cutting tool _____
    d. It doesn't need to be held _____

5. What part(s) of the printing press can most likely cause injury when the press is in use?

    a. The turning spokes _____
    b. The rollers _____
    c. The bed _____
    d. The press table _____

Note to student: When you have finished this part of the test, notify your teacher and arrange to demonstrate the use of the linoleum block printing tools.

Figure 16.

Multiple choice questions are quick to evaluate and can be used effectively because there are specific answers. When student judgment is required, short answer or essay tests are more effective. Combining multiple choice with observation increases the effectiveness of the test.

   3. Prohibit participation in activities unless the tests have been satisfactorily passed.
- Maintain complete records of the health and safety activities that are part of the regular art program.
  1. Keep copies of all inventory lists, condition reports, requests for elimination of room hazards, student tests, permission slips and information on allergies.
  2. Keep lesson plan copies indicating that health and safety instruction was planned and actually provided in each class session.
  3. Maintain a complete description of the artroom health and safety program, plans for using warning and information signs and copies of the constitution of student health and safety committees and minutes of any meetings.

LIABILITY INSURANCE

There is little question that even if a teacher meticulously follows all these suggestions for avoiding litigation, there still remains the possibility that someone may file a law suit charging negligence. Because the laws in a number of states provide protection from litigation against school districts (known as the principle of *sovereign immunity*), it may actually be illegal for the district to provide liability insurance for its employees. The reasoning is that since the district can't be held liable, it cannot spend district funds for liability insurance.

Each teacher should make an effort to find out the liability coverage that may be provided as a part of employment. If there is none, seek other sources for it. Most professional organizations make liability insurance available to members at reasonable cost (for example, the National Art Education Association [NAEA] has such insurance available to its members). Determine if the coverage pays legal fees as well as any judgments that might be rendered. Do not be shy about seeking substantial coverage: judgments in tort actions often reach the hundreds of thousands of dollars, and legal fees can be very heavy.

A good teacher, careful in health and safety instruction, will take this extra step to insure against ruin. Liability insurance will not ease the emotional pain a teacher feels from knowing a student may have been handicapped for life as a result of a classroom accident. But the lack of adequate insurance may make a tragic situation even worse.

RECORDS INUNDATION

No teacher wants to add to an already heavy record-keeping burden and art teachers seem to be in a special class when it comes to finding reasons to avoid paper work. There is no question that filling out forms and maintaining files strike most teachers as busy work and an eminently avoidable waste of time. This attitude should not prevail against health and safety program records.

Maintaining a safe workplace to protect oneself from litigation ought to be reason enough for teachers to keep the required records. If not, charges of irresponsibility, if not negligence, are most certainly in order.

However, there are ways to keep this task reasonable. Once the initial information has been collected, only a small amount of time will be required to keep everything current.

- Assign one file drawer strictly for health and safety materials. Divide the drawer into three separate sections:
  1. One should contain all material relating to the overall health and safety program, such as a general plan, the organization of health and safety committees and statements about reporting procedures for health and safety activities.
  2. One should be used for folders holding blank forms to make inventories and condition checks, tests, requests for information, permission slips to be signed and reports to be forwarded to the school administration.
  3. One should hold individual files containing completed forms in all the categories mentioned above. There should also be folders for copies of any reports that have been submitted to anyone about any aspect of the health and safety program.
- Use student help to make inventories and condition checks. However, be sure to verify their observations and initial their reports to indicate agreement with their judgment.
- Regularly and habitually include comments on health and safety instruction in lesson plans; keep those plans indefinitely.

- When classes have been completed at the end of each semester or year, take all of the folders with records pertaining to the students, tie them into a bundle, label them clearly, and store in the school archives. If the school does not have such a place, take them home and store them where they can be found easily. There would be little reason to keep such records if the only concern was injury from accidents in the artroom. But, with the increasing awareness of chronic illness resulting from exposures to chemicals in art processes, it would be well to maintain these records for a much longer period of time.

Being the defendant in negligence litigation is a very real possibility for any art teacher. Even if the record keeping is tiresome and time-consuming, it should not be considered too much trouble. In this regard, there are two pieces of advice which every art teacher should heed:

Be a careful teacher who is aware of health and safety hazards in the artroom, who instructs students carefully, tests skills and knowledge adequately and monitors behavior constantly.

Be able to prove it.

APPENDIX

Health and Safety Equipment and Material Sources

Supply company catalogs, in addition to being sources of equipment, provide excellent general information about health and safety. The following suppliers' catalogs are comprehensive and include nearly all equipment that might be useful in an art classroom. They are a quick and valuable resource for the art teacher.

DIRECT SAFETY COMPANY

7815 South 46th Street, Phoenix, AZ 85044.

The catalog describes a wide variety of protective clothing including gloves, glasses and goggles, respirators, masks and hearing protection. Among other things, this company also distributes first aid gear, flammable storage cabinets and containers, eyewash and emergency shower equipment and safety signs. Catalog is in color with clear informative descriptions of items.

HENRY'S SAFETY SUPPLY CO

P.O. Box 30277, Billings, MT 59107

P.O. Box 540, Casper, WY 82602

P.O. Box 3168, Gillette, WY 82716

1215 Elk Street, Rock Springs, WY 82901

2900 E. Broadway, Warehouse #12, Bismark, ND 58501

14252 West 44th Ave. Golden, CO 80403

Henry's mammoth catalog (over 600 pages) includes health and safety equipment for eye and face protection, respiratory, hearing and head protection, first aid supplies, eye wash and shower equipment, hand and foot protection and safety signs and markers. Supplies for other safety needs, not specific to art classrooms, are also included. Illustrations are in black and white, but item descriptions are thorough and educational.

LAB SAFETY SUPPLY

P.O. Box 1366, Janesville, WI 53547

This comprehensive catalog contains illustrations of health and safety supplies in all categories important to art teachers. There are also sections on educational aids and safety books. Many of the books are too technical and specialized for art teachers but could be of use to school district health and safety officials.

NATIONAL SAFETY COUNCIL

444 North Michigan Avenue, Chicago, IL 60611

The general materials catalog lists a variety of printed educational materials useful in the artroom. Also included are films and videotapes on safety and instructional slide sets.

BIBLIOGRAPHY

Barazani, Gail C. *Safe Practices in the Arts and Crafts; A Studio Guide.* New York: College Art Association of America, 1978.

Carnow, Bertram. "Natural Disease-Unnatural Cause," address, Health Risks in the Arts, Crafts, and Trades Conference: Chicago, April 2, 1981

Clark, Nancy, Thomas Cutter, and Jean-Anne McGrane. *Ventilation A Practical Guide.* New York: Center for Occupational Hazards, 1984.

Doull, John, Curtis D. Klassen, and Mary O. Amdur, eds. *Toxicology.* New York: Macmillan Publishing Co., 1980.

Florio, A.E., W.F. Alles, and G.T. Stafford. *Safety Education.* New York: McGraw-Hill Book Company, 1979.

Flygare, Thomas. *The Legal Rights of Teachers.* Bloomington, IN: The Phi Delta Kappa Foundation, 1976.

Gatti, R.D. and D.J. Gatti. *Encyclopedic Dictionary of School Law.* West Nyack, NY: Parker Publishing Co., Inc., 1975.

Hemeon, W.C.L. *Plant and Process Ventilation.* New York: The Industrial Press, 1963.

Loeffler, J.J., ed. *Industrial Ventilation.* 18th Edition, Lansing, MI: American Conference of Governmental Industrial Hygienists, 1984.

McCann, Michael. *Artist Beware.* New York: Watson-Guptill Publications, 1979.

_____. *Health Hazards Manual for Artists.* Third Edition. New York: Nick Lyons Books, 1985.

McCarthy, Martha M. and Nelda H. Cambron. *Public School Law.* Boston: Allyn and Bacon, Inc., 1981.

McElrory, Frank E., ed. *Accident Prevention Manual for Industrial Operations.* Chicago: National Safety Council, 1969.

NIOSH. *Preventing Health Hazards from Exposure to Benzidine Congener Dyes.* Washington, D.C.: U.S. Department of Health and Human Services, 1983.

_____. *Welding Safety.* Washington, D.C.: Government Printing Office, 1980.

Peterson, L.J., R.A. Rossmiller, and M.M. Voltz. *The Law and Public School Operation.* 2nd Edition. New York: Harper and Row Publishers, Inc., 1978.

Pittaro, Ernest M., ed. *The Compact Photo Index.* Dobbs Ferry, NY: Morgan and Morgan, Inc., 1977.

Qualley, Charles, "Art Hazards Survey," *School Arts,* Vol. 83, No. 8, April, 1984, pp. 47–48.

Qualley, Charles and Marc Swadener, "The Art Hazards Survey: Initial Results," *School Arts,* Vol. 84, No. 7, March, 1985, pp. 41–45.

Seeger, Nancy. *A Ceramist's Guide to the Safe Use of Materials.* Chicago: The Art Institute of Chicago, 1982.

———. *A Painter's Guide to the Safe Use of Materials.* Chicago: The Art Institute of Chicago, 1982.

———. *A Photographer's Guide to the Safe Use of Materials.* Chicago: The Art Institute of Chicago, 1983.

Shaw, Susan. *Overexposure: Health Hazards in Photography.* New York: Friends of Photography, 1983.

Siedlecki, Jerome T. "Potential Hazards of Plastics Used in Sculpture." *Journal of the National Art Education Association.* Vol. 25, February, 1972.

INDEX